Contents

Preface

The idea that some plants can be used beneficially for food or for medicine, while others can be harmful if eaten or even touched, is part of ancient folklore. One of the earliest written accounts of plant poisoning is in the Old Testament where an incident that took place about 900 BC is recorded. At a time of food shortage, when 'herbs' were being collected, the introduction of 'gourds' from a 'wild vine' into a pot of soup caused those eating it to exclaim that there was 'death in the pot'!* Despite the great increase in our knowledge of the subject since that time, it remains difficult to define a poisonous plant. In many cases it can be stated with certainty that a particular plant is poisonous, because of the frequency or severity of incidents associated with it, but to state that another plant is definitely not poisonous is too bold an assertion, as isolated instances of poisoning by previously unsuspected plants are still reported from time to time. In addition, there are variations among the plants themselves and differences in susceptibility among animal species and among individuals within those species. It must be emphasized that the toxicity of cultivated species and varieties of a poisonous wild plant is often not known. Plants are, in fact, not frequent causes of poisoning in Britain, partly because the few dangerous ones are well known and therefore avoided, and partly because (with the notable exception of bracken) there are few areas in the country where extensive growth of poisonous wild plants occurs.

The purpose of this book is to provide information on the plants (including fungi) found in Britain that are known to have had adverse effects on people or animals, either here or abroad. It has been written in the simplest possible style, and is intended as a layman's guide to the subject. The information presented will, however, be a useful source of quick reference for doctors, veterinarians and farmers, particularly as coverage of the subject has been made as complete as possible by including fungi, garden and house plants as well as the many wild ones and a few crops.

Wherever possible, the plants are referred to by their common names, these being based on the *Flora of the British Isles* (1987) by A. R. Clapham, T. G. Tutin and D. M. Moore and *English Names of Wild Flowers* (1986) by J. G. Dony, S. L. Jury and F. H. Perring; the latter is the recommended list of the Botanical Society of the British Isles. In order to avoid ambiguity and to enable precise identification, the Latin names are also used, mainly in accordance with the *Flora* mentioned above, *A Dictionary of Flowering Plants and Ferns* (1973) by J. C. Willis and *Handwörterbuch der Pflanzennamen* (1984) by R. Zander. The main part of the book is devoted to accounts of some 80 plants and 20 fungi that are the most likely or the most dangerous causes of plant poisoning in Britain,

*2 Kings 4, 38–40

5

although most of the plants mentioned also occur in other countries. Alphabetical order has been used for the families into which the plants are grouped, and also for the genera and species within each family. For each plant or group of plants, a brief description is followed by details of poisonous substances, symptoms of human and animal poisoning and recommendations for treatment (where appropriate). The botanical descriptions are included for general guidance, but should, in conjunction with the illustrations, be adequate for identifying the plants. Much of the veterinary and some of the medical information is a simplified form of that presented in the authors' previous publication *Poisonous Plants in Britain and their effects on animals and man* (1984; MAFF Reference Book 161). The coverage of the subject has been expanded, in the present book, to include more plants that could be involved in human poisoning, particularly garden and house plants. In the extensive searches through medical and veterinary literature, on which these books are based, information was also collected on poisoning by other plants related to those in the main text, on plants of lesser or dubious toxicity and also on those well known to be poisonous in other countries, but found only infrequently here. This information has been included in lists, a special feature of the book, covering a further 160 plants and 15 fungi, and giving brief notes about each. Most of the plants and fungi in the main section and a few of those in the lists are illustrated. Contact with many plants can produce a skin reaction in certain individuals sensitive to them. Although some reference is made to such reactions, the complex problem of skin sensitivity to plants is not covered in detail.

It is our hope that this book will help to make people more aware of the potential dangers of plants to themselves, their children and their animals, and thus reduce the number of unpleasant or tragic incidents that occur from this source every year.

We wish to thank Dorothy Elliott for her careful and prompt typing of the manuscript, and all of our other colleagues at the Commonwealth Bureau of Animal Health for their interest and encouragement, particularly Mike Hails BSc, Dip Agric Econ, whose annotated bibliography *Plant Poisoning in Animals* (published by CAB International, Wallingford) was such a valuable source of references. We should like to acknowledge the help of Margaret Davidge and other members of the library staff of the Central Veterinary Laboratory who obtained for us much useful information. We should also like to thank our long-suffering friends and especially our families who have been both patient and helpful during the long hours we have devoted to the preparation of this book.

MARION R. COOPER
ANTHONY W. JOHNSON
CAB International Bureau of Animal Health,
Central Veterinary Laboratory,
Weybridge, Surrey.

List of common names and illustrations

Plants

This list includes all the plants dealt with in detail in the main text (most are illustrated). For alternative common names of these plants and also for other poisonous plants not having such detailed entries, the index at the back of the book should be consulted. An annotated list of the less important plants can be found on pages 93–110.

Fungi

The fungi in this list are described in the main text of the book; other poisonous fungi are listed on pages 124–125.

Photograph acknowledgements

We are most grateful to Dr. Hugh Baillie, who provided most of the photographs; some were from his extensive collection, but many were taken especially for this book. The other photographs were kindly provided by Dr. Roy Watling and the Royal Botanic Garden, Edinburgh (photos 90, 91, 92, 95, 96, 99), Sylvia Berrett (6, 12, 49, 52), A-Z Botanical Collection Ltd (53, 55, 68, 71, 77), Dr. Derek A. Reid (88, 89, 98), Dr. Alan Beaumont (78), Dr. J. C. Forbes and the School of Agriculture, Aberdeen (80), and ADAS (85, photographed by John R. Morrison, Harpenden Laboratory).

Introduction

If you stand and look around in many gardens or almost anywhere in the countryside it is generally easy to see at least two or three of the plants mentioned in this book. Poisonous plants are common and can be found in most households, gardens, hedgerows, fields and woods. There are also many poisonous mushrooms and toadstools growing in the wild. Despite this, surprisingly few instances of plant poisoning are reported in either people or animals. When such poisoning does occur it is generally found that there was some special circumstance present that contributed to why that particular plant, plant part or fungus was eaten. Appreciation of these contributory factors will help in recognizing potentially dangerous situations, so that these can be avoided and possible cases of poisoning prevented.

Contributory factors in human poisoning

Children and berries

Young children exploring the world around them at the crawling and toddling stages are particularly likely to pick up small objects, such as berries, from the ground and put them into their mouth. Older children and even adults are attracted by berries and fruits on plants and may mistakenly think they can be eaten. The commonest enquiry received by doctors about the toxicity of plants is from anxious parents whose child has swallowed some (often unidentified) berries.

Mistaken identification

The increasing popularity of gathering plants growing wild in the countryside as a source of 'natural' food can lead to poisonous plants being eaten instead of, or together with, edible ones. Particularly dangerous errors can be made with mushrooms, which are notoriously difficult for the non-expert to distinguish from one another with certainty; some can produce very severe or even fatal poisoning. The Umbelliferae family, which includes familiar edible vegetables such as parsnips, carrots and celery, also contains rather similar, but highly poisonous, wild plants, of which the most dangerous in Britain are cowbane, hemlock and hemlock water dropwort. Various poisonous bulbs, such as those of bluebells and daffodils, have been eaten in mistake for onions. People making their own herbal medicines or preparing herbal teas have mistakenly included either poisonous plants or medicinal plants in quantities sufficient to have toxic effects.

11

Hallucinogens

The use of some plants and mushrooms known to have hallucinogenic effects has led to poisoning in two ways:

1. too much of the hallucinogen being taken, with the result that coma and even death have occurred;
2. incorrect identification, with a more toxic species than intended being used.

Contributory factors in animal poisoning

Feed shortage

This can occur as a result of seasonal fluctuations or adverse weather conditions such as drought or snow. For example, in autumn when cattle and horses may be short of green feed on pasture, they will eat acorns. In heavy snowfalls when there is little other feed, animals tend to eat any available green foliage, such as rhododendron, cherry laurel or yew, especially if the branches are brought within their reach by being weighed down with snow. When grazing animals do not have sufficient grass in their fields, whatever the reason, they are likely to break out and gain access to gardens and woodland, where there may well be poisonous plants.

Hay and silage

Some poisonous plants, such as buttercups, lose their toxicity in feed preserved in this way. Others, such as ragwort, are still toxic but lose their unpalatability, so becoming more likely to cause poisoning.

Pasture management

Poor pasture management and overgrazing can lead to the predominance of poisonous plants such as buttercups, ragwort and bracken.

Weed control

Poisonous plants previously ignored by grazing animals may be eaten very readily after application of weed-killers or if pulled up or cut and left lying on the ground.

Garden refuse disposal

Thoughtless disposal of garden rubbish, such as hedge trimmings from box, laburnum, cherry laurel, privet, rhododendron, or yew, and other household waste, such as rhubarb leaves, is an important cause of sporadic cases of poisoning. If poisonous material of this sort is thrown into fields, the curiosity of animals is aroused and they may well eat it.

Hedging and drainage

These operations can expose poisonous roots, such as those of cowbane and iris.

Boredom

Dogs and cats shut in a house alone may chew house plants, some of which can cause poisoning.

Inappropriate feeding

Dogs and cats have been poisoned by being fed left-over food containing onions, pigs by being given discarded plums, pet rabbits by cherry laurel leaves, and zoo animals by foliage or fruits picked from nearby ornamental shrubs. Dogs have been poisoned by chewing laburnum and oleander sticks that have been thrown for them to retrieve.

Unfamiliar surroundings

Animals introduced into new surroundings are at risk from poisonous plants previously ignored by other animals already used to that environment.

Toxicity of poisonous plants

Some plants, such as yew, oleander and cowbane, are highly toxic and small amounts can produce fatal poisoning. Other plants, such as bracken and ragwort, have to be eaten in quite large amounts for a prolonged period to cause poisoning. Where the quantity eaten is an important factor in determining whether a plant is likely to cause poisoning, it is only the grazing and browsing animals (horses, cattle, sheep and goats) that eat enough to give rise to signs of toxicity.

Not all the parts of a so-called poisonous plant are necessarily poisonous. For example the seeds within the fruits of the yew are highly toxic, and sudden death can occur if they are chewed, yet the surrounding red flesh can be eaten without any harmful effects at all. Rhubarb stalks are edible when cooked as a dessert, but the leaves should never be eaten. The toxic constituents (poisonous substances) are not necessarily distributed uniformly throughout a plant but may be present in greater concentrations in certain parts. The concentration of these substances can also vary with the stage of growth and growing conditions of the plant.

Poisonous substances

There are numerous chemical compounds recognized as being responsible for the toxic effects produced by poisonous plants. Some of these were given names many years ago, often based on the Latin name of the plant in which they were found, e.g. hederin, from holly *(Hedera helix)*. Since then, some of these have been shown to be a mixture of compounds, and, although the chemical identity and structural formulae of the more important of the compounds have been determined, there are still many for which these are not known. Even where the individual chemical substances have been isolated and identified, it is frequently not understood precisely how they produce their effects in man or the larger mammals and their toxic doses have not been calculated for the different animal species likely to be poisoned.

Some, but not exhaustive, information is given in the main text of this book on the poisonous substances found in the plants described. This can be useful in two ways:

1. as an indication of the type of treatment that can be used in some cases, e.g. cyanide poisoning;
2. as a guide to the effects of other plants containing the same substance.

Traditionally the poisonous substances in plants have been classified as:

   alkaloids
   glycosides (cardiac, cyanogenic, goitrogenic, and saponic)
   nitrates-nitrites
   oxalates
   phenols
   photosensitizing agents
   proteins, peptides and amino acids
   tannins
   volatile oils

Toxic substances that belong to all of these classes are present in one or more of the plants mentioned in this book, although most of those found in plants in Britain are either alkaloids or glycosides. The prime function of these appears to be to defend plants against attack by insects and micro-organisms; they are probably only incidentally poisonous to mammals.

There can often be considerable variation in the toxicity of plant populations and even individual plants within a species. Some of this variation arises when the plants in question are threatened by, or under attack from, specific pests. As a defence they produce various chemical substances that can be poisonous to people and farm and pet animals, in addition to deterring or killing the pest. Some cultivated garden and indoor varieties of plants tend to be less toxic than those of the same species growing in the wild; a few are more toxic. Season, weather conditions and the nature of the soil can also influence plant toxicity.

In addition to variation in the toxin content of plants there is variation in the susceptibility of different species of animals and also among individual animals of the ·same species. The considerable variation in the dose that produces a toxic effect in the different animal species is dependent not only on the size of the animal and the structure and functions of the digestive system but also on the way the various species break down the poisonous substance once it has been absorbed.

The differences in the toxicity of plants and even in their various parts, as well as the differing susceptibility of animals, make it difficult to define what is a poisonous plant. The plants considered in this book are those which, when any part is eaten or in some cases touched, can give rise to a departure from the normal health of man or domestic animals. They can be broadly classified as fungi (mushrooms and toadstools) and wild, garden, and house plants. In addition, the incorrect use of some food plants or excess feeding of farm animals with some agricultural crops grown in this country can also have harmful effects (see page 91).

Symptoms of plant poisoning

The mouth, then the stomach and the rest of the digestive system are usually the first parts of the body to be affected when poisonous plants are eaten. Some plants that have very irritant sap, such as dumb cane, mezereon, cuckoo pint, spurges and black bryony, give rise at once to soreness, reddening and even blistering of the lips and mouth. With most plants the first sign of poisoning may be nausea, abdominal pain and vomiting. It must be remembered, however, that not all animals can vomit. Ruminants (cattle, sheep, goats) vomit only in exceptional circumstances, such as when poisoned by rhododendron, *Pieris* and lily of the valley; horses do not vomit. In many cases, vomiting eliminates the poisonous substances and prevents any further development of poisoning. Elimination of the poisonous substances is also promoted by diarrhoea, another very common reaction to eating poisonous plants. Constipation is a feature of poisoning by only a few plants such as oak, ash and deadly nightshade.

After absorption into the body from the digestive tract, the poisonous substances pass first to the liver where many are broken down and lose their toxicity. Liver damage can also occur however, and is found, in particular, after poisoning by plants, such as ragwort, which contain pyrrolizidine alkaloids. Other poisonous substances, such as those in the onion family, have a direct effect on the blood cells and cause anaemia. In poisoning by oxalate-containing plants, such as rhubarb and fat hen, there is a reduction in the calcium content of the blood, resulting in signs of weakness, staggering and inability to stand. The kidneys can be damaged by poisonous substances passing through them, as occurs in poisoning by the fungus *Cortinarius* and by oxalate-containing plants.

The poisonous substances of some plants sensitize the skin to ultraviolet light, so that signs of severe sunburn appear on unpigmented or hairless parts of the skin after exposure to bright sunlight. Such photosensitizing plants are St. John's wort, buckwheat and giant hogweed.

Signs of plant poisoning attributable to effects on the nervous system are probably second in frequency only to signs of digestive disturbances. Some plants, such as cannabis and morning glory, and also some fungi, particularly the psilocybin-containing mushrooms, produce changes in behaviour and mental state. In cases of severe poisoning by a number of plants there are convulsions and unconsciousness.

In some types of poisoning that are fatal, the immediate cause of death is heart failure as a result of the toxin acting directly on the heart; foxglove, oleander and yew have this effect.

Diagnosis

A definite diagnosis can be made fairly confidently if it is realized that a sick person or animal has eaten parts of a known poisonous plant. It must be remembered, however, that there is a considerable range in time between eating a poisonous plant and the appearance of symptoms; with certain plants the effects occur almost immediately, whereas with others it may be up to 48 hours before they become apparent. Grazing animals may eat even quite large quantities of some plants for weeks or months before signs of poisoning appear.

The most common difficulty is knowing whether or not the plant or plant part that has been eaten is poisonous, as in the case of a child who has put a berry in its mouth and the worried parent cannot identify it. Provided that what has been eaten is not a wild mushroom and that there are no immediate signs of toxicity, it is only necessary to watch the child carefully for a couple of days. If symptoms appear, and medical attention is required, any berries or parts of the plant, as well as any vomit, should be taken, along with the patient, to help the doctor make a diagnosis.

The symptoms produced by eating most poisonous plants are the same as those that occur very commonly in many other types of digestive system disturbances and infectious diseases. In fact, the vast majority of cases of nausea, vomiting, abdominal pain and diarrhoea are not due to eating poisonous plants. Poisoning by plants and fungi cannot be diagnosed on symptoms alone.

Farm animals can eat some poisonous plants for prolonged periods before signs of disease become evident; occasionally these appear only when the animals no longer have access to the plants responsible. In such cases, diagnosis can be very difficult and requires veterinary experience and laboratory investigations. In animals it is sometimes possible to make a definite diagnosis only after a post-mortem examination, when plant parts may be found in the stomach. Chemical analysis is generally of little help in establishing a diagnosis.

Treatment

Prevent any further intake of the poisonous substance by taking out any plant parts still in the mouth and stopping further access to the plant.

Obtain expert advice from a doctor or veterinary surgeon, as appropriate, if there is any suspicion of serious poisoning. They have the training and experience to assess the problem and decide on a course of action:

1. to initiate treatment themselves;
2. to request specialist advice from a poisons centre;
3. to refer the case to a hospital.

Specific antidotes to plant toxins are available for only a few types of poisoning, such as those caused by cyanides, nitrites and oxalates. There are, however, two basic principles to follow when treating all types of plant poisoning:

1. the removal of poisonous material still in the digestive tract (stomach and intestines) or on the skin;
2. the maintenance of the essential functions of the body so that it can respond to and deal with the poisonous substances and the damage caused.

Methods of removing the poisonous material from the digestive tract include the induction of vomiting, stomach washouts, the administration of activated charcoal, and the use of appropriate purgatives. These procedures should be carried out under professional supervision. If a rash or blisters develop on the skin after contact with the sap of a plant, the affected areas should be washed immediately with warm water.

Other important measures contributing to recovery include treatment to alleviate symptoms and also supportive nursing to aid the natural detoxification processes of the body.

Plant names

The common names of plants, such as foxglove, old man's beard and Solomon's seal, are often very attractive, and can sometimes give an idea of the nature of the plant, as in the case of bluebell, or where it grows, as in the case of the small mushroom called dung roundhead; however, they do not necessarily identify a plant accurately. More than one plant may be called by the same common name, or conversely, more than one common name can be used for the same plant; common names differ in various parts of a country and especially from country to country, each language having its own name or names for a plant. For these reasons a system of classification of plants (and animals) has been developed, the one in use today being based largely on the work of the Swedish scientist Linnaeus (1707–1778). In this system Latin is used throughout, and related plants are grouped together. The names of plant families end in -ae (usually -eae and often -aceae), such as Gramineae or Buxaceae, and contain one or many smaller groups, called genera (genus in the singular); each genus contains one or more individual plants which are called species. The species name applies to only one plant, that is, it is specific. There may be plants with minor differences within one species, particularly among cultivated plants. These are called varieties, and may or may not have a Latin name. Varieties may exist in the wild or may be developed by selective cultivation, when they are often called cultivars. It is customary to use initial capital letters for families and genera, and small letters for species and varieties; genera and species are usually printed in italics. When naming a plant, the genus is given first, followed by the species and then the variety (if any), e.g. the potato, in the family Solanaceae, is called *Solanum* (genus) *tuberosum* (species) followed by variety, such as 'King Edward'. Despite the system outlined above, the naming of the plants is continually being revised in the light of new work on classification, and discrepancies will still be found. Plants are occasionally moved from one family or genus to another or even given completely new names. In some cases there is a lack of agreement among the various recognized authorities, resulting in plants being referred to by different names in different books, or classified differently, as in the case of onions and related plants that are sometimes placed in the Alliaceae family and sometimes in the Amaryllidaceae or Liliaceae families.

Poisonous plants

Many plants in this family, such as onions *(Allium cepa)*, leeks, chives, shallots and garlic, are grown for culinary use, as they give a distinctive flavour to cooked food; they can also be eaten raw. The plants differ considerably in the shape of their leaves and underground parts, but all have a characteristic smell if cut or crushed. Wild garlic *(Allium ursinum)*, crow garlic *(Allium vineale)*, and onions themselves are the members of this family that have been reported to cause poisoning in Britain.

Ramsons *Allium ursinum* (photo 1)
Wild Garlic

This spring-flowering woodland plant is common throughout Britain in damp, shady places, where it may be the dominant ground-cover plant. It is not immediately recognizable as a member of the onion family. It has bright-green leaves that are elliptical in shape and pointed at the tip, 10–25 cm (4–10 in) long and about 5 cm (2 in) wide; as in other *Allium* species, the veins run parallel along the length of the leaf. The flowers are white, larger than those of onions and form a loosely clustered head, often about 30 cm (12 in) above the ground.

Another wild member of this family is the crow garlic *(Allium vineale)*. This plant is less common than formerly, because weed-killers have been applied where it grew, on road verges and farmland.

● POISONOUS SUBSTANCES All parts of the plants contain n-propyl disulphide and other related volatile compounds, which cause the breakdown of red blood cells, with consequent anaemia.

● POISONING Human poisoning has not been reported after eating any wild or cultivated member of the onion family, although soreness and watering of the eyes occur in the presence of cut or crushed plant parts, particularly the bulbs of onions.

It is inadvisable to give food containing appreciable quantities of onions to household pets or to allow them to eat raw onions as both dogs and cats have been poisoned in this way: after eating onion soufflé, dogs became lethargic and anaemic, with vomiting and frequent passage of reddish or dark urine; cats that ate onion soup or raw onions became anaemic.

Feeding large quantities of discarded onions or onion waste to farm animals can cause poisoning, although sheep, in particular, seem to enjoy them. Poisoning has also resulted from eating the foliage and flowers of ramsons or crow garlic. Cattle and horses seem to be more susceptible than sheep or goats. Affected animals become weak and anaemic and produce dark, blood-stained urine. They may stagger as they move, or become paralysed. The pulse becomes weak and breathing more rapid and there is often loss of weight and appetite. The breath of the animals smells of onions, and both milk and meat can be tainted.

There is no specific treatment; animals generally recover gradually after removal of onions from their diet.

• **NOTE** Care should be taken not to confuse stored onions with other bulbs, such as daffodils, which can cause poisoning if eaten.

AMARYLLIDACEAE

This family contains many garden and house plants, some of which are called 'lilies' and may be included mistakenly in the Liliaceae family. Poisoning has occurred most frequently when the bulbs, particularly those of daffodils (see below), have been confused with onions. Other members of the family (such as those listed on page 93) can cause poisoning resembling that produced by daffodils.

Daffodil *Narcissus* species (photo 3)
Garden Narcissus; Jonquil

Wild daffodils *(Narcissus pseudonarcissus)* remain in only a few areas of Britain, but there are many cultivated varieties and hybrids. These common spring flowers develop each year from bulbs below the ground. Narrow leaves, up to 30 cm (12 in) long, appear first and persist until after flowering. Wild daffodil flowers are yellow, but the cultivated ones are white or shades of yellow or orange. Each flower has a central trumpet, with a ring of pointed, triangular lobes at its base.

• **POISONOUS SUBSTANCES** The whole plant, and particularly the bulb, contains alkaloids (lycorine and galanthamine) and a glycoside (scillaine).

• **POISONING** When the bulbs have been mistaken for onions and eaten, either raw or cooked, symptoms including dizziness, stomach pains, nausea, vomiting and diarrhoea have developed shortly afterwards. In more severe poisoning there may be trembling, convulsions and paralysis. Vomiting has occurred in children who have eaten a few leaves, and there is also a report of a four-year-old child who died after sucking a narcissus stalk. Recovery, however, is usually complete in a few hours without any treatment being necessary. Those who pick and pack the flowers are liable to develop dermatitis, probably caused partly by the irritant effects of the sap and partly by an allergic reaction.

Animals rarely eat these plants, although, during the food shortage in the Netherlands in the Second World War, some cattle died after being given narcissus bulbs to eat. A tortoise which ate four daffodil leaves lost its appetite and became constipated and listless; it died 11 days later.

In severe cases it may be necessary to induce vomiting or remove stomach contents.

● NOTE Care should be taken not to confuse harvested onions with lifted daffodil bulbs; most cases of daffodil poisoning have been the result of such mistakes.

APOCYNACEAE

In addition to the highly toxic oleander (see below), this family includes some house plants that can cause poisoning (see page 94).

Oleander *Nerium oleander* (photo 4)

This flowering shrub is a native of southern Europe, but is hardy enough to survive most winters out of doors in the warmer parts of Britain; it is also grown here as a glasshouse plant. When left untrimmed, oleander can grow to 3 m (10 ft) in height and width. The leaves are elongated and pointed, with a prominent midrib. The shrub blooms profusely in late spring or early summer, when large clusters of flowers develop; these are usually shades of red or pink, but there are also some white and yellow varieties.

● POISONOUS SUBSTANCES Every part of the plant contains glycosides that affect the action of the heart in the same way as the glycosides in foxglove. The toxicity remains after drying or boiling.

● POISONING It has long been recognized that this is an extremely dangerous plant; eating it can be fatal, and even smoke from a fire on which it is burning is toxic. In other countries, skewers of oleander wood used in cooking meat have led to fatal poisoning. Recently a person died after drinking herbal tea made by boiling oleander leaves (mistaken for eucalyptus). There is an immediate burning sensation in the mouth and a bitter taste that often prevents further consumption of the plant, although even small amounts can cause severe poisoning. In a few hours there is numbness of the tongue, abdominal pain, nausea, vomiting and diarrhoea (sometimes with blood), and a rapid pulse. Other symptoms include dilatation of the pupils and visual disturbances, yellow and green colours and patterns being seen around objects. The serious effects of oleander poisoning develop a little later when there is a slow, weak, irregular pulse and a fall in blood pressure. It is these effects on the rhythm and functioning of the heart that can lead to death. Contact with the plant, and especially with the sap, can cause soreness and blistering of the skin.

Although animals do not usually eat oleander, isolated instances with symptoms similar to those in human poisoning have been reported in a wide variety of animals, including horses, cattle, goats, monkeys, a sloth, a bear and swans.

Urgent professional treatment is required as poisoning by oleander can be fatal.

AQUIFOLIACEAE

The most common holly in this country (*Ilex aquifolium*) has occasionally caused mild poisoning (see below). The toxicity of other species and varieties is not known.

Holly *Ilex aquifolium* (photo 6)

Holly is a common evergreen shrub or small tree which grows wild throughout Britain, except on very wet soils. It is the most common shrub below tree level in some woods, as it tolerates shade. There are many other species and garden varieties, some of which are variegated. Holly is immediately recognizable by its thick, dark-green leaves, 4–6 cm (1½–2½ in) long. They are glossy above and have sharp points at the tip and also at the end of each projection of their very wavy margin. The leaves on some twigs, particularly flowering ones and those on old trees, are more or less oval with few or no points. In late spring, clusters of small white flowers appear; these develop into shiny green berries that turn bright red in winter, when they feature prominently in Christmas decorations.

● POISONOUS SUBSTANCES In the middle of the last century several glycosides, such as ilicin, were described and named after the plant, but little is known either about them or about the effects of other possible toxins present (saponins, triterpene compounds).

● POISONING It is not uncommon for children to eat holly berries, especially when brought indoors at Christmas time. They are not dangerously poisonous if only a few are eaten, but can cause persistent vomiting and diarrhoea; even two berries can produce nausea. It has been suggested that eating 20–30 berries could be fatal, but no reports have been found to confirm this.

Little information is available on poisoning in animals, but in a recent incident two foals were found dead after eating holly leaves when there was little other feed available.

If a child eats more than two or three holly berries, vomiting should be induced as soon as possible.

ARACEAE

Cuckoo pint (*Arum maculatum*) a wild plant (see below), and several of the most popular house plants available in Britain belong to this family. The common and scientific (Latin) names of many of the house plants are often incorrectly used, with the various names being interchanged and applied to different plants, resulting in some confusion. Some of the more common of these are described below, and details of poisoning given for one, the dumb cane (*Dieffenbachia*), which appears to cause the most severe reactions. It should be stressed, however, that most (perhaps all) of the house plants in this family can cause similar symptoms, although they vary considerably in severity. Others are listed on page 94.

Cuckoo Pint *Arum maculatum* (photos 7 and 8)
Lords and Ladies; Wild Arum

Cuckoo pint grows in shady places in most parts of Britain, except northern Scotland; it is commonly found in woods, hedgerows and gardens. The leaves grow early each spring from the underground tuber which has white flesh but is brown outside. Each leaf has a long stalk and a blade that is triangular or shaped like a barbed arrow. The blade is up to 20 cm (8 in) long, fairly dark green, and has a network of veins; in some varieties there are irregular brownish-purple spots on the upper surface. The flowers and associated structures are characteristic of this family, and have an erect yellowish-green sheath, 15–25 cm (6–10 in) long, that opens widely on one side to reveal a central, dull-purple cylindrical structure, up to 10 cm (4 in) long. The fruits develop below this as a closely packed group of berries that are green initially but ripen to a bright reddish orange. At this stage the rest of the plant dies down, leaving only the conspicuous fruits on the pale-green flower stalk.

• POISONOUS SUBSTANCES Calcium oxalate crystals, present in all parts of the plant, are most probably responsible for the toxicity, although there are many references to a 'volatile acrid substance' called aroin (or similar names), the precise nature of which is not known. The toxicity of the berries is variable. Drying or boiling reduces, but does not completely destroy, the toxicity of this plant.

• POISONING Although the leaves and roots of the plant have caused isolated cases of poisoning, most cases occur as a result of the attractive, ripe berries being eaten, particularly by children. The berries have a sweet taste, but quickly cause a sensation of burning and soreness of the mouth, lips and throat. If more than a few berries are eaten, more serious signs of poisoning may develop: nausea, vomiting, abdominal pain, muscular cramps, dilatation of pupils, dizziness, irregular pulse and even coma and death. Severe poisoning is, however, unusual, because the burning experienced in the mouth is a deterrent to eating large amounts.

Under normal circumstances, animals also rarely consume sufficient of the plant to cause more than mild poisoning, but when there is little else to graze, both leaves and berries have been eaten, sometimes in considerable quantities. After eating the leaves, cattle have shown excessive production of saliva, digestive-system disturbances, unsteadiness, convulsions and coma; some have died. Sheep have developed similar symptoms, with profuse diarrhoea; abortion in horses has also been attributed to the plant.

Professional treatment is required in all but mild cases.

Elephant's Ear *Caladium* species
Several other related plants also have the common name Elephant's Ear.

This is a popular ornamental house plant on account of its spectacular leaf colouring. In common with other members of the family, *Caladium* has long-stalked, broadly spear-shaped leaves that may be up to 30 cm (12 in) long. Depending on the variety, the leaves may have smooth or wavy margins and mottling, spotting or irregular blotching with shades of pink, red, cream or white; in some the leaves are green, but the veins are red or whitish. There are hundreds of named varieties available. These can produce a type of poisoning similar to but less severe than that caused by *Dieffenbachia* (see below).

Dumb Cane *Dieffenbachia* species (photo 9)

This popular house plant is grown for its foliage; the flowers, partially enclosed in a greenish sheath, are less attractive and seldom develop in this country. In its natural habitat, South America and the West Indies, the plant may grow up to 2 m (just over 6 ft) high, but as a house plant it rarely exceeds 60 cm (2 ft). The upright stem is partly sheathed by the bases of the leaf stalks, giving a somewhat jointed appearance. As a continuation of the stalk, the leaves have a prominent midrib, particularly apparent on the underside. The young leaves are loosely curled along their long axis, but when expanded they are broad and oval, tapering at the tip and towards the stalk. They can be up to 40 cm (16 in) long, but in many specimens, they are less than 30 cm (12 in). Several species of *Dieffenbachia* are common as house plants; there are many varieties and some hybrids. These are distinguishable by the characteristic markings on the upper side of the leaves. There may be white or yellowish lines following the main veins, or an irregular pattern of whitish blotches.

• POISONOUS SUBSTANCES It is generally agreed that the constituent causing most of the symptoms is calcium oxalate, present in the sap as needle-like crystals, but a protein-splitting enzyme may also be involved.

• POISONING Although the whole plant is poisonous, poisoning usually results from the leaves being chewed. A sharp, pricking sensation, sometimes likened to chewing glass splinters, is experienced in the mouth, and it is probable that mechanical damage by the sharp crystals precedes poisoning by the oxalates. An intense, burning pain, accompanied by reddening and swelling of the mouth, tongue and throat occurs very quickly after chewing the plant; the swelling may be so severe that the throat becomes partly blocked, restricting breathing. In some cases the voice is partially or completely lost for a while – hence the common name, dumb cane. It is said that the plant has been used as a form of torture, and to stop prisoners from speaking. Symptoms are usually restricted to the mouth and throat, but occasionally nausea and vomiting have been reported. Care should be taken when tending these plants, as eye injuries, lasting for up to four weeks, have resulted from sap squirting into the eye during trimming or the removal of old leaves.

Animals are affected similarly if they chew the leaves of *Dieffenbachia*.

Washing with warm water is recommended for removing sap from the skin and mouth; professional advice should be sought if the eyes are affected or if any part of the plant is chewed or swallowed.

• NOTE This plant is a potential danger to both children and domestic pets and should be kept out of their reach.

Cheese Plant *Monstera deliciosa* (photo 10)

Swiss Cheese Plant; Mexican Breadfruit and many others

In its natural state *Monstera* is a woody climber, but in this country, where it is a popular house plant, it grows like a small shrub, sometimes attaching itself to supporting sticks by the aerial roots with which it climbs. The leaves are large, sometimes exceeding 30 cm (12 in) long, and are broad and pointed. They grow on long stalks that have a sheathing base. A few leaves, especially those near the base of the plant, have a smooth edge and no holes, but most are deeply and irregularly indented from the edge and perforated with several large elongated, oval holes or splits. It is for its unusual foliage that *Monstera* is grown, but older, mature plants sometimes produce sweet-smelling, yellowish flowers, rather like arum lilies. *Monstera* can produce a type of poisoning similar to but less severe than that caused by *Dieffenbachia* (see above).

Elephant's Ear *Philodendron* species

The common name, Elephant's Ear, is also used for other plants in this family.

In Britain *Philodendron* is a popular house plant, grown for its attractive foliage. Although some plants climb readily by attaching themselves to suitable supports by means of aerial roots produced from the stems, others grow as small, more compact shrubs. There are a great many varieties, most with heart-shaped or spear-shaped leaves that are dark green and glossy. They can produce a type of poisoning similar to but less severe than that caused by *Dieffenbachia* (see above).

Arum Lily *Zantedeschia* species

Calla Lily (mainly in the USA). Occasionally called Richardia.
These plants are not true lilies, which are members of the Liliaceae family.

These are grown as house plants or for cut flowers. Most varieties have long-stalked, tough, shiny, spear-shaped leaves up to 30 cm (12 in) long; they are usually uniformly dark green, but some are flecked with white. The flowers are very small and crowded together on an erect, cylindrical structure surrounded by a simple white or yellow sheath that is an attractive, conspicuous feature of the plant.

The flamingo flower (*Anthurium*, photo 5) is similar to the arum lily. It has longer, more oval leaves and a bright red sheath around the thin, cylindrical structure bearing the flowers; this is also bright red, usually curved or twisted and projecting from the sheath. At the base of the flower, attractive, coloured (usually red) fruits, like berries, sometimes form. Both *Zantedeschia* and *Anthurium* can produce a type of poisoning similar to but less severe than that caused by *Dieffenbachia* (see above).

ARALIACEAE

The ivy *(Hedera helix)* that is commonly found growing wild in Britain has long been regarded as poisonous. The toxicity of garden species and varieties is not known.

Ivy *Hedera helix* (photo 11)

This evergreen climber is common throughout most of Britain, and is very tolerant of shade. It has tough, woody stems, and near the base of older plants there may be a small trunk, with well-developed bark. Densely packed, short roots that grow along the stems attach the plant to other trees, walls or fences or it may spread along the ground. The leaves are dark green, often with lighter-green veins, and are sometimes tinged purple. Those of the climbing stems have three to five triangular lobes; those of the flowering stems are not lobed, but oval, with a pointed tip. The small, yellowish-green flowers appear in autumn in rounded clusters; spherical black berries develop later, and may persist until the following spring.

• POISONOUS SUBSTANCES Triterpenoid saponins, from which toxic substances called hederins are formed, are present in all parts of the plant.

• POISONING Human poisoning most frequently involves the berries; these have an unpleasant, bitter taste and usually not many are eaten. Symptoms are, therefore, rarely serious and are limited to a burning sensation in the mouth and throat, although there are some old reports of vomiting, difficult breathing, convulsions and coma. Contact with ivy can cause skin reactions of varying severity. Symptoms range from a mild rash to blistering and swelling in sensitive persons; such sensitivity to ivy is not uncommon.

Poisoning in animals can be more serious, as large quantities of leaves and berries are sometimes eaten. Ivy poisoning has occurred in cattle, sheep, deer and dogs. The symptoms include vomiting, diarrhoea, excitement, staggering and paralysis; affected animals sometimes appear to have abdominal pain. Their breath may have the smell of crushed ivy leaves, and milk may be tainted. Poultry have died after eating ivy seeds. The practice of giving cattle a few ivy leaves as a 'tonic' does not do any harm.

Treatment of human poisoning is usually unnecessary, and full recovery can be expected within a few days; vomiting should be induced if large numbers of berries have been eaten. Animals with severe symptoms require veterinary attention.

• NOTE Ivy cut from trees or pulled off walls is a potential danger to animals.

ASPIDIACEAE

In this family only the male and buckler ferns *(Dryopteris* species) are generally regarded as poisonous (see below). A much more common fern that can cause serious poisoning is bracken *(Pteridium aquilinum)* in the Dennstaedtiaceae family (see pages 41-42)

Male Fern and Buckler Fern
Dryopteris species (photo 12)

There are several of these ferns and some hybrids in Britain. The male fern *(Dryopteris filix-mas)* is one of the most abundant. It is a tall, perennial fern, with erect, unbranched leaves (fronds) up to 1.5 m (5 ft) long, arising from one or more crowns at ground level. The stalks are covered with brownish-orange scales, and carry rows of very deeply divided, fairly bright-green leaflets. The bottom leaflets are longer than those near the tip of the leaf. There are closely packed, spore-bearing structures on the back of some leaves. Unlike those of bracken, the leaves of these ferns may stay green throughout the winter.

• POISONOUS SUBSTANCES A complex mixture of substances, called filicin, is found at the bottom of the stalks and in the underground stem.

• POISONING There are no reports of human poisoning by the wild species or other *Dryopteris* ferns used as house plants.

Poisoning has been reported only in cattle, and seems to occur initially when green feed is scarce, but animals may persist in eating the plants even after adequate feed is available. Affected animals may stagger and become constipated, but the chief effect is blindness, with widely dilated pupils that do not respond to light. Some animals regain their sight, while others remain permanently blind, although recovery is complete in every other respect.

BERBERIDACEAE

This family contains many cultivated species and varieties of *Berberis* and the closely related genus *Mahonia* (see page 95); some have become naturalized and may be found growing wild. In the past these shrubs were often planted for their fruits, which were eaten cooked in various ways; now they are grown chiefly for their attractive flowers and foliage. Little is known about the toxicity of wild barberry or that of the individual cultivated forms, but a general account is given below.

Barberry *Berberis* species (photo 13)

It is doubtful if barberry *(Berberis vulgaris)* is a truly native plant of Britain, although it is occasionally found, apparently growing wild, in hedgerows or scrub. *Berberis* species are much branched shrubs, growing 1–3 m (3–10 ft) high. The small leaves, which often develop attractive autumn colours before falling, are broadly oval or pointed, and up to 4 cm (1½ in) long, depending on the variety. Beneath each cluster of leaves is a group of sharp spines less than 2.5 cm (1 in) long. The flowers are yellow (often orange or reddish in cultivated forms) and grow in small clusters. In late summer, rectangular or cylindrical, reddish-orange, sour-tasting berries develop.

• POISONOUS SUBSTANCE An alkaloid, berberine, is present, mainly in the bark, but also in the seeds of some species.

• POISONING In common with the berries of many other plants, those of the wild barberry and its many cultivated varieties give rise to numerous enquiries concerning possible harmful effects, particularly in children. The berries of wild barberry are not poisonous and can even be used for preserves, but those of some cultivated forms contain appreciable quantities of alkaloids and could cause mild poisoning. There have been reports of vomiting and diarrhoea in people handling the wood or taking medicinal preparations containing berberine. Penetration by *Berberis* spines can give rise to inflammation and blistering of the skin.

No reports have been found of *Berberis* poisoning in animals.

BORAGINACEAE

There are reports of poisoning by a number of plants in this family (see note below), but most attention has been paid to the *Symphytum* species, particularly comfrey *(Symphytum officinale)*, used in herbal preparations.

Comfrey *Symphytum officinale* (photo 14)

This plant is often found beside rivers and streams, in damp places or on road verges throughout the country, particularly in the south. Comfrey is a coarse, hairy, greyish-green plant with large lower leaves, 15–25 cm (6–10 in) long from the tapered point to where they join and run down the stem. The flower stalk is up to 1.2 m (4 ft) tall and bears erect clusters of pinkish, purple or creamy-white flowers; in the bud stage the top of the stalk bends downwards.

• POISONOUS SUBSTANCES Pyrrolizidine alkaloids are present in comfrey and also in other plants of the same family, with the alkaloid content in comfrey being highest in the young leaves. The alkaloids persist in dead plants. Some species, such as rough comfrey *(Symphytum asperum)*, accumulate nitrates, from which toxic nitrites are formed.

• POISONING There are no reports of human poisoning by comfrey, and medicinal preparations of the plant and comfrey tea are still made. Their use, however, has diminished following publicity given to experiments in which rats developed liver tumours after having been given large quantities of comfrey extract for a long period.

At pasture, domestic animals are unlikely to consume enough comfrey to poison them, but if the plant is fed to them, there is the risk of poisoning; pigs that were fed on rough comfrey developed nitrate-nitrite poisoning, with difficult breathing and bluish discoloration of the mouth.

Veterinary advice should be sought, because a specific treatment is available for this type of poisoning.

• NOTE Other plants of the family found in Britain have been responsible for poisoning only in other countries where they are widespread. Their alkaloids have given rise to poisoning resembling that caused by ragwort. In horses, hound's tongue *(Cynoglossum officinale)*, present in hay, caused liver disease and subsequent damage to unpigmented skin after exposure to light (photosensitization). Horses that ate purple viper's bugloss *(Echium plantagineum,* photo 15) became lethargic and uncoordinated; blindness and death occurred in some cases.

BUXACEAE

Box *(Buxus sempervirens)* is the only member of this family that has caused poisoning in Britain; the toxicity of others, several of which are cultivated in gardens, is not known.

Box *Buxus sempervirens* (photo 16)

This evergreen shrub has grown wild in Britain at least since the 13th century, when there were references made to it in the early history of Box Hill, in Surrey. Although in the wild state box is abundant in some areas of chalk and limestone, it is limited in its distribution to a few places in southern England, where it often grows with yew, giving dense shade beneath taller, usually beech, trees. It is planted, however, in most of the country as an ornamental shrub or hedging plant. The shrub is usually 3–5 m (10–16 ft) high, but may grow up to 9 m (about 30 ft). The bark is grey and the twigs are slightly angled and hairy. They bear numerous small, leathery, oval leaves, up to 2.5 cm (1 in) long, which are paler beneath than on the top; their tips and sides often curve downwards. In late spring, whitish-green flowers develop in clusters consisting of one female flower and several male flowers.

• POISONOUS SUBSTANCES Several related alkaloids, previously thought to be a single substance and named buxine, are present in all parts of the plant. The alkaloids remain active in foliage that has been cut or accidentally broken from the shrub.

• POISONING Box is not a plant that people would find attractive to eat, and no cases of human poisoning have been reported.

Animals rarely eat box, possibly because of its bitter taste and disagreeable odour when bruised, but poisoning has occurred in horses, cattle and pigs, usually after they have browsed garden hedges or trimmings. The digestive system is affected, with pain, vomiting and diarrhoea. In severe cases there may be difficulty in breathing, loss of coordination, convulsions, coma and death. Box is poisonous for fish and should not, therefore, be placed in their tanks.

Severe cases of poisoning require professional treatment.

CANNABACEAE

In this family the only plant whose toxicity has been studied in detail is the hemp plant *(Cannabis sativa)*, the source of the notorious drug named after it.

Cannabis *Cannabis sativa*
Hemp

Cannabis plants are large, erect and usually unbranched, growing up to 2 m (7 ft) high in the course of the year. The leaves are rough to touch and are divided into usually seven narrow, elongated lobes. The male and female flowers arise in the axils of the leaves and are borne on separate plants. The male flowers are in loose clusters; the females are less conspicuous, occurring in short spikes with only the feathery stigmas protruding. In some parts of the world, cannabis plants are grown because their stems provide a good quality textile fibre (hemp). In Britain the plant is covered by the Misuse of Drugs Act, and at present it is illegal to grow it. The development of new varieties with negligible drug content, but good stem fibre, is in progress. Cannabis plants sometimes grow wild in waste places where the seed has been discarded.

● **POISONOUS SUBSTANCES** The resinous material that exudes from the plants contains tetrahydrocannabinols, which are potent drugs that, even in small quantities, can induce changes in mental state and behaviour, and, in larger quantities, coma and death. The resin is found in its highest concentration in the female flowers, and is still active when the plants have been dried. The name of the plant, cannabis, is one of the names applied to the drug prepared from it; other names are hashish, marijuana, hemp and pot.

● **POISONING** People who take or smoke cannabis expect it to have a relaxing effect, with enhanced perception of enjoyment; this is often accompanied by poor concentration and reduced ability to perform tasks requiring mechanical skills. The effects depend on the amount and frequency of consumption. Large amounts can result in extremely unpleasant mental experiences and physical side effects: delusions and misconception of surroundings, nausea, trembling, headaches and even coma.

Pet animals, especially dogs, occasionally gain access to and are poisoned by cannabis preparations used by their owners. They may develop muscular weakness, staggering, sleepiness and vomiting; most recover within 24 hours. Cannabis plants, when growing, are generally avoided by animals, perhaps because of their bitter taste. Horses, however, have died after eating the plant.

CAPRIFOLIACEAE

The members of this family that are known to be poisonous belong to the genera *Sambucus* and *Symphoricarpos*. Of these, dwarf elder (*Sambucus ebulus*), elder (*Sambucus nigra*) and snowberry (*Symphoricarpos rivularis*) have been involved in cases of poisoning. The toxicity of other garden species is not known. Plants such as honeysuckle (*Lonicera*) and *Viburnum* species (see page 95) have been suspected of causing poisoning, but are of low or doubtful toxicity.

Elder *Sambucus nigra* (photo 17)

Elder is a common deciduous shrub, occasionally a tree, that grows in waste places, hedges and scrub in most parts of Britain, except northern Scotland. Some elders are cultivated in gardens. The bark is grey and deeply furrowed on older parts. The wood is not strong, as there is a large area of pith in the branches and twigs. The leaves consist of several, usually oval, pointed leaflets arranged in pairs on either side of the stalk. Many small, creamy-white flowers form in flat-topped clusters in summer and develop into characteristic hanging bunches of dark reddish-black, spherical fruits, usually considerably less than 1 cm (½ in) across.

Dwarf elder or danewort *(Sambucus ebulus)*, although a related plant, is not a woody shrub like the elder, but has similar leaflets and flowers, sometimes pinkish white, and black fruits in autumn.

• POISONOUS SUBSTANCES *Sambucus* species contain a substance that causes vomiting and diarrhoea, and also cyanide-producing glycosides; all parts are poisonous.

• POISONING Human poisoning is most likely to occur from eating raw berries; even a few berries could lead to nausea, vomiting, stomach pains, diarrhoea, weakness and coma. In 1983, fruit juice, prepared by crushing elder berries, with their leaves, caused symptoms of poisoning within 15 minutes in a party of people in a remote area of California; the eight most severely affected had to be flown to hospital by helicopter but all recovered quickly.

Presumably because of its bitter taste, animals generally do not eat *Sambucus*, but symptoms similar to those of human poisoning have been seen in pigs that ate the leaves. In one outbreak 14 of 50 pigs died; they had rapid breathing and heart rate, trembling and paralysis.

Professional advice should be sought if the symptoms are severe.

• NOTE Heating destroys most of the toxicity, and flowers and berries used for wine making or in pies are not harmful.

Snowberry *Symphoricarpos rivularis* (photo 18)

Snowberry was introduced into Britain as a garden shrub, but is now found in many places growing wild, spreading into fairly dense, bushy thickets by means of suckers from the roots. The bushes are 1-3 m (3-10 ft) high, with yellowish twigs that bear small, oval leaves, 2-4 cm (¾-1½ in) long. They are a dull, light green; some leaves may persist through the winter. The small pink and white flowers develop in a tight cluster, and characteristic waxy, dull-white, round berries appear in autumn. Berries in a cluster may vary in size from 0.5-1.5 cm (¼-½ in) in diameter.

• **POISONOUS SUBSTANCES** The toxicity of *Symphoricarpos* has been attributed to several of its constituents, but no definite information is available.

• **POISONING** Eating the berries has caused vomiting, diarrhoea, dizziness and, in severe cases, unconsciousness. Generally, when only three or four berries have been eaten, there are no symptoms, but there is one recent report of a child who vomited and became slightly dizzy and drowsy after eating only three berries. Although this plant has gained quite a reputation for being dangerously poisonous, this is based mainly on a much quoted report of poisoning of children in Norfolk in 1885. There have been very few recent incidents.

There are no reports of poisoning in animals.

CELASTRACEAE

The member of this family that is known to cause poisoning is spindle (*Euonymus europaeus*). Other *Euonymus* species are cultivated in Britain, but their toxicity is not known.

Spindle *Euonymus europaeus* (photo 19)

This branched, rather stiff shrub or small tree is fairly common in woodland and scrub, mainly on chalk or limestone soils. The bark is smooth and grey; the young twigs are green and square in section. The leaves are elongated, oval and pointed at the tip; they turn red in autumn. The leaf stalks and sometimes the stems are tinged red. The flowers are insignificant, up to 1 cm (⅓ in) across, and have greenish petals. The fruits are 1–1.5 cm (⅓–½ in) across, and have deep-pink, fleshy lobes that split apart to reveal the bright-orange covering of the seed. Several spindles are cultivated for their autumn colours and attractive fruits.

• **POISONOUS SUBSTANCES** All parts of the shrub contain glycosides, which affect the heart, and an agent that causes digestive system disturbances, but very little is known about these substances.

• **POISONING** The parts most likely to cause human poisoning are the fruits. Symptoms appear 8-16 hours after eating, when vomiting, abdominal pain and diarrhoea occur. In more severe cases these can become persistent, and there may be disturbances in blood circulation with drowsiness, convulsions, and loss of consciousness.

Animals seldom eat this plant and few cases of poisoning have been reported; eating young shoots, however, has caused abdominal pain, constipation and death in horses, and severe diarrhoea in sheep and goats. Professional advice should be sought in severe cases.

CHENOPODIACEAE

Some well-known edible plants such as sugar beet and fodder beet belong to this family; under certain circumstances some of them have caused poisoning when fed to animals (see Crop plants, page 91). A few wild species, particularly fat hen *(Chenopodium album)* and orache *(Atriplex* species*)*, can cause photosensitization (see below).

Fat Hen *Chenopodium album* (photo 20)

This is a common wasteland plant, but is also found on poor arable land as a weed among crops. The form and size of the plant are variable; the usual height ranges from 30–60 cm (1–2 ft), the stems are single or branched and may have a reddish tinge, the leaves are diamond shaped or oval with a pointed tip, and their edges are toothed or smooth. In late summer, tiny flowers develop in small, tightly packed clusters at the top of the branches. They are the same lightish-green colour and have the same characteristic powdery appearance as the young leaves.

• POISONOUS SUBSTANCES Oxalates in fat hen are responsible for poisoning in grazing animals. A substance causing people to become sensitive to sunlight is also present and remains active even after boiling.

• POISONING This is likely to occur only if large amounts of fat hen are eaten. At times of food shortage, as in eastern Europe during and after the Second World War, people have eaten *Chenopodium* raw in salads or cooked as a vegetable. Exposure of the skin to sunlight after eating the plant results in severe skin damage, with swelling and blistering, and ulcers that are slow to heal. Human poisoning, with similar symptoms, has been recorded after eating orache *(Atriplex)*.

Cattle and sheep that have grazed pastures containing large amounts of fat hen become listless, with staggering movements, shallow breathing, and weak heart beat; milk production decreases. Severely affected animals may be unable to stand, lose consciousness and die. In cattle, fat hen poisoning resembles milk fever.

Veterinary advice should be sought if symptoms are severe.

COMPOSITAE

Ragwort *(Senecio jacobaea)*, a member of this family, is one of the most important causes of plant poisoning in farm animals in Britain. Other *Senecio* species found in this country contain varying concentrations of toxic substances similar to those found in ragwort, but generally these species do not grow in such situations or in such an abundance that poisoning is likely to occur. Some wild and garden plants in the Compositae are also potentially toxic (see page 96).

Ragwort *Senecio jacobaea* (photo 21)

This plant is common on wasteland, roadsides and in poor pastures. From a flat rosette of leaves at ground level, a stiff, erect, often reddish-tinged flowering stem grows, sometimes branching part way up. The plant varies in height according to where it is growing, but is normally 30 cm–1 m (1–3 ft) tall. The leaves are tough, dark green, and very irregularly and deeply indented, giving a ragged appearance; those at the top of the plant are not stalked and tend to lie close to the stem. The closely packed heads of small, bright-yellow flowers are a conspicuous feature of ragwort in summer.

● **POISONOUS SUBSTANCES** There are several pyrrolizidine alkaloids present in the whole plant; they remain active in hay and silage.

● **POISONING** Although herbal preparations made from ragwort have had some undesirable effects, the plant itself is not a direct cause of human poisoning. The toxic alkaloids may be present in the milk of poisoned animals or in honey made from the plant, but the risk of poisoning from these sources appears to be negligible in Britain.

Ragwort is one of the commonest causes of plant poisoning in farm animals, its alkaloids causing serious damage to the liver. Cattle and horses are the most frequently affected. In general, animals avoid ragwort while grazing, unless other pasture plants are scarce, as, for example, during a drought. Under such conditions, some animals may develop a strong preference for the plant and continue to eat it even when better pasture becomes available. Most cases of ragwort poisoning occur after the plant has been eaten in dried grass, hay or silage. The animals may not show symptoms until they have been eating ragwort for several weeks, or months, or even when they no longer have access to the plant, but, if large amounts of ragwort are eaten in a short time, the symptoms may appear within a few days. The first signs of poisoning are abdominal pain and diarrhoea, with persistent straining. The general condition of the animals deteriorates and they may appear jaundiced; exposure to bright sunlight may lead to soreness affecting unpigmented areas of skin as a result of the liver damage (photosensitization). Animals become agitated, aggressive, and tend to keep walking; they may press their heads against walls or fences and are apparently unaware of their surroundings. Severely affected animals appear blind and may become uncoordinated and partially paralysed before losing consciousness and dying. Goats are often said to be resistant to ragwort poisoning, but prolonged feeding with the plants has led to symptoms similar to those in cattle, with severe liver damage. Although toxic alkaloids are present in goats' milk, the kids are apparently unaffected. Sheep are less susceptible than goats, and may even be used to clear pasture of young ragwort plants, but they may still suffer some liver damage. The effects of ragwort poisoning are often noticed for the first time when animals are under stress, such as pregnancy or when they have infections. Because of the non-specific nature of many of the symptoms (involving general loss of condition), ragwort poisoning is not easy to diagnose, but if suspected, it is obviously necessary to remove animals from access to the plant at pasture or in feed; once the liver has been severely damaged, however, recovery is unlikely.

Professional advice is needed for the treatment of animals, and also for the control of ragwort on pasture.

● NOTE Clearing pasture of ragwort is essential for the safety of grazing animals but can be a difficult and expensive operation. In the past, hand-pulling was carried out, but herbicide application is now the method of choice. Uprooted plants and those recently treated with weed-killer are, however, particularly attractive to animals, so treated pasture should be left for at least two weeks before allowing animals on to it.

CONVOLVULACEAE

In this family some varieties of morning glory (cultivated *Ipomoea* species) are poisonous (see below), as are the wild parasitic dodders (*Cuscuta* species) that occur in some parts of Britain (see list, page 98).

Morning Glory *Ipomoea* species (photo 22)

These climbing plants, related to bindweed, are found only in greenhouses and gardens, as they are rarely hardy enough to survive a winter in Britain. The smooth, twisting stems may be up to 3 m (10 ft) long, and bear pointed, heart-shaped leaves and showy, trumpet-like flowers. These are of many different colours, depending on the species, but most are red, pink or blue, sometimes with white. Each flower lasts only a day or two, but many are produced; seeds are not necessarily formed.

● **POISONOUS SUBSTANCES** The hallucinogenic alkaloid, d-lysergic acid amide (LAA), also called ergine, is present in varying amounts in the seeds of some varieties. It has a similar action to the drug LSD, but is less powerful. Other alkaloids are also present.

● **POISONING** The ability of morning glory seeds to induce psychic changes has been known for centuries by Mexican Indians, who have used the plant in religious rituals. Much more recently, particularly since the 1960s, its use and abuse by drug takers to induce hallucinations have been increasing. There is considerable variation in the alkaloid content of the seeds of different *Ipomoea* species, and the effects they have are unpredictable; they can last for many hours and may be very unpleasant and frightening. In addition to altered perception of colour, shape, sound and time, there may also be nausea, vomiting, diarrhoea, mental confusion and disorientation.

Animals do not usually eat *Ipomoea*, but cattle, sheep and goats have been poisoned by eating the growing plant. Digestive-system disturbances, convulsions and coma have been reported.

Professional advice should be sought if symptoms are severe.

CRUCIFERAE

This family contains some wild plants that occasionally cause poisoning (see page 98), and many familiar food plants that can, under certain circumstances, have toxic effects (see Crop plants, page 91). Both the leaves and roots of horse radish can be harmful (see below).

Horse Radish *Armoracia rusticana* (photo 23)

This perennial plant is grown for use as a condiment, but has become naturalized in many places and can be seen on waste ground, road verges and agricultural land. Horse radish has a thick, branched, fibrous rootstock, from which large, coarse leaves develop in spring. They are bright green, toothed at the edges, 30–45 cm (12–18 in) long, and 10–15 cm (4–6 in) wide. The basal leaves have long stalks, but those on the stem have only short or no stalks. The stems are up to 1 m (3 ft) high, and a much branched cluster of very small white flowers develops at the top in summer.

● **POISONOUS SUBSTANCE** All parts of the plant contain sinigrin, a gluco-sinolate.

• **POISONING** Horse radish sauce, prepared by grating the white flesh of the root, has a sharp, hot taste and is a traditional accompaniment to roast beef. It has, however, occasionally produced digestive upsets in children. Contact with the sap of the plant can cause soreness of the eyes and skin.

Animals rarely eat horse radish, but it has caused the death of cattle and horses that have grazed the leaves, and of pigs fed with hotel refuse containing the grated root. They all showed signs of severe abdominal pain before death.

CUCURBITACEAE

This family contains many familiar food plants such as cucumbers, vegetable marrows and pumpkins, but also includes white bryony *(Bryonia dioica)* a poisonous climbing plant that grows wild in Britain (see below).

White Bryony *Bryonia dioica* (photos 24 and 25)

This plant is often thought to be related to black bryony *(Tamus communis)* but the latter is in a different plant family (Dioscoreaceae); both are poisonous.

White bryony is found throughout most of Britain, but less commonly in the north. It has a very large root that has the same unpleasant, acrid smell as the rest of the plant when cut. Every spring, long trailing stems, often several metres (yards) long, grow from the root and climb, by attachment of coiling tendrils, to other plants. The leaves are lightish green, 5–10 cm (2–4 in) across and have three or five broadly pointed lobes. On both leaves and stems there are small, stiff hairs that make the plant somewhat coarse to touch. Clusters of small, greenish-white flowers, about 1 cm (⅓ in) across, develop at the base of the leaves; male and female flowers grow on separate plants. As the leaves yellow and begin to die back in autumn, round, dull-red berries develop on the female plants.

• **POISONOUS SUBSTANCES** There is little definite information about the nature of these; a glycoside (bryonin) and an alkaloid (bryonicine) are among the substances incriminated.

• **POISONING** The berries are the parts of the plant most likely to be eaten, especially by children. Less than ten berries can produce repeated vomiting; larger numbers can, in addition, cause stomach pains, diarrhoea (with blood), dizziness and difficulty in breathing. Eating the roots has also caused human poisoning.

Farm animals are occasionally poisoned by eating bryony growing in hedgerows, but it is when the roots are exposed and eaten that most cases of poisoning occur. There is severe digestive disturbance, with diarrhoea and breathing difficulty; cows may stop giving milk for several days. A herd of 40 cows that had eaten white bryony roots, dug out when a pipeline was being laid, collapsed within a few hours. Their bodies were cold and their eyes sunken; they all lost consciousness and died. Horses poisoned by white bryony may sweat profusely and produce excessive amounts of urine as well as having diarrhoea; they may become uncoordinated and have convulsions. Ducklings have died after eating the plant, and fatal poisoning has also occurred in poultry that have eaten the berries.

Professional advice should be sought if more than mild symptoms appear.

CUPRESSACEAE

Within this family, cypresses belonging to the genus *Cupressus* are known to be poisonous (see below); other cypresses are included in the genus *Chamaecyparis*. Some reports of poisoning in animals refer only to 'cypress' and it is not clear which genus is involved.

Cypress *Cupressus* species (photo 26)

Cypresses are evergreen coniferous trees, not native to Britain, but often planted here singly or as hedge plants and windbreaks. Several species and varieties are grown; some have attractive yellowish foliage, and some are very fast growing. All will withstand regular trimming, but if left to grow, they become tall, slender trees, up to 24 m (80 ft) high, with side branches usually close together and almost down to ground level, so that the reddish-brown trunk is scarcely visible. The leaves are small, deep green, triangular and scale-like, growing close to each other and to the stem of the twigs, which are branched in one or more planes, depending on the species. The female cones are small, rounded structures, usually less than 1 cm (⅓ in) across. They are made up of tightly overlapping scales that become woody and open slightly at maturity. The male cones are smaller and sometimes brightly coloured.

● POISONOUS SUBSTANCE This has not been identified.

● POISONING Cypress is most unlikely to be eaten, and there are no reports of human poisoning.

Cattle have been poisoned by eating cypress foliage, with symptoms developing in one to two weeks. The animals become weak and listless, with staggering movements; the eyes are often sunken and some animals may die. Cypress is particularly dangerous for cows in late pregnancy, as they are liable

to abort; those that recover produce little milk initially.
- **NOTE** Animals should not be allowed access to felled cypress trees, branches or hedge trimmings.

DENNSTAEDTIACEAE

Bracken *(Pteridium aquilinum)* is one of the commonest causes of plant poisoning of livestock in Britain. It is sometimes classified in the Hypolepidaceae or Polypodiaceae family.

Bracken *Pteridium aquilinum* (photo 27)

Bracken is a very common fern that grows throughout Britain, except in wet places and limestone country. In many areas it is spreading into valuable pasture, where it rapidly becomes dominant in the existing grassland. Chemical control is extremely expensive because of the very large areas now occupied by bracken and, particularly in hilly country, eradication by ploughing is impracticable. In addition to loss of pasture, the increase in bracken is highly undesirable because of its toxicity to grazing animals.

Bracken is a tough, strongly growing fern. It spreads by creeping underground stems from which the new leaves (fronds) grow in late spring. They unroll as they develop, to form large, branched leaves 30 cm–2 m (1–7 ft) or more high, depending on the growing conditions. The leaves are subdivided into smaller, deeply indented leaflets, some of which have brown, spore-bearing structures on their undersides. In autumn the leaves become brown and often remain lying on the ground throughout the winter.

- **POISONOUS SUBSTANCES** Several constituents are poisonous, including a cyanogenic glycoside (prunasin) that is, however, usually present in harmless quantities, an enzyme (thiaminase) and a heat-stable antithiamine factor that lead to thiamine (vitamin B_1) deficiency in horses and pigs, and a carcinogen (ptaquiloside) responsible for diseases in cattle and sheep. Work is still in progress on elucidating the carcinogenic activity of bracken. Some of the toxins of bracken remain after drying.

- **POISONING** In countries where the human consumption of young bracken fronds is customary, this has been associated with the occurrence of tumours of the digestive system. There is also the possiblity of a bracken carcinogen (an agent inducing cancer) being acquired indirectly through milk, meat and the water supply; these aspects are still being investigated.

The consumption of bracken gives rise to a variety of responses, depending on the species of animal involved and differences in their susceptibility to the poisonous constituents of the plant: 'bracken staggers' in horses,

41

haemorrhagic 'bracken poisoning' in cattle, bladder tumours (enzootic haematuria) and digestive-system tumours in both cattle and sheep, and 'bright blindness' in sheep.

Signs of thiamine deficiency develop in horses (bracken staggers) and pigs, but not in ruminant animals such as cattle and sheep in which thiamine is produced in the rumen. In horses, signs of poisoning appear one to two months after they have started to eat bracken, when staggering, muscle twitching, irregular heart beat, loss of appetite and loss of condition develop. In severe cases, these are followed by convulsions and death. Poisoning by bracken rarely occurs in pigs because they do not normally have access to it, but when it does occur there may be sudden death or, in less severe cases, loss of appetite, vomiting, and heavy breathing.

'Bracken poisoning' in cattle occurs after they have been eating considerable quantities of the leaves or underground stems of the plant for several weeks; symptoms then develop quickly and include the appearance of blood in the faeces and urine and discharges (sometimes with blood) from the eyes, nose and mouth. These characteristic haemorrhages are followed by progressive weakness; similar symptoms have occasionally been seen in sheep.

When cattle and sheep have been eating small quantities of bracken over a long period, there is loss of blood in the urine, with the development of tumours in the bladder (enzootic haematuria). Attacks of increasing severity can occur before death. This disease has only recently been associated with eating bracken. In addition to tumours of the bladder, it has been shown that eating bracken can also lead to tumour formation in the digestive system of cattle and sheep.

In sheep, the consumption of bracken for long periods can lead to a form of permanent blindness in which the eyes remain bright and clear (bright blindness).

If any of these conditions is suspected, the animals should be removed from bracken-infested land and veterinary advice sought; thiamine deficiency responds well to treatment.

DIOSCOREACEAE

The only member of this family that grows wild in Britain is black bryony (*Tamus communis*), a poisonous climbing plant.

Black Bryony *Tamus communis* (photos 28 and 29)

This plant is not related to white bryony (*Bryonia dioica*), which belongs to another plant family (Cucurbitaceae); both are poisonous.

Black bryony is common in southern England, but less so from the Midlands northwards. The root is an irregularly shaped, blackish tuber, from which smooth, unbranched stems grow in spring. These coil around each other and around other vegetation, fence wires, etc. and can be several metres (yards) long. Dark-green, glossy, pointed, heart-shaped leaves with long stalks are present at intervals along the stem; from the base of the leaves small clusters of greenish-yellow flowers grow in summer. Separate groups of male and female flowers are present on the same plant, the males having longer stalks. Shiny, green, spherical berries, sometimes up to 1 cm (⅓ in) across develop in late summer; they become black when ripe.

• POISONOUS SUBSTANCES Over the years, several substances have been suspected, but the needle-shaped calcium oxalate crystals found in the plants appear to be responsible for most of the symptoms. With the exception of the young shoots, all parts of the plant contain these crystals; they are abundant in the roots and berries.

• POISONING Black bryony poisoning is similar to that caused by *Dieffenbachia* (page 25) and *Arum maculatum* (page 23).

The berries are particularly attractive to children, in whom they can cause severe blistering and burning of the mouth and digestive system, resulting in vomiting and diarrhoea. Rubbing of the skin with the cut surface of the black, tuberous underground parts of the plant causes swelling, redness and burning. Eating a large quantity of the tuber can be fatal, although severe poisoning is rare.

Animals seldom eat black bryony, but three horses died after pulling the plant from a hedge and eating it. They had severe abdominal pain and profuse sweating before death.

Washing with warm water is recommended to remove the irritant sap from the skin and mouth; professional advice should be sought if symptoms are severe.

EQUISETACEAE

The horsetails *(Equisetum* species), of which there are several in Britain, are the only members of this family; some are troublesome weeds.

Horsetail *Equisetum* species (photo 30)
Mare's Tail

The field horsetail *(Equisetum arvense)* and the marsh horsetail *(Equisetum palustre)*, found throughout the country, are the ones most likely to cause poisoning in animals.

Horsetail is a perennial plant with a creeping underground stem from which green, jointed, upright stems grow in spring. The stems, up to 80 cm (32 in) but often less than 45 cm (18 in) high, are hollow or partly hollow and have narrow longitudinal grooves. At each joint on the stem, a ring of fine, similarly jointed branches emerges, giving the plant a somewhat delicate appearance, although it is harsh to touch. The leaves are inconspicuous, appearing just above the joints as a small sheath with a toothed upper edge. Separate brownish stems, usually without branches, also develop, but are far less numerous than the green ones; at the top of each of these is a cone-like structure in which spores develop.

● POISONOUS SUBSTANCES There are several potentially poisonous substances in horsetails, the one most likely to cause problems being an enzyme, thiaminase (also found in bracken), that destroys vitamin B_1 (thiamine), resulting in symptoms of vitamin B_1 deficiency. The toxicity remains after drying and storage.

● POISONING This coarse plant is not attractive as a source of food and is not a likely cause of human poisoning.

While it is growing, animals tend to avoid horsetail, presumably because its high silicate content makes it rough and unpalatable. Poisoning is most likely to occur when horsetail is present in hay or bedding. Even as little as 5% of the plant in hay is enough to cause problems. Symptoms may develop quickly or be delayed for several weeks after eating the plant. Horses are the most severely affected, with loss of weight, loss of condition, weakness, muscular twitching and staggering, which can progress to paralysis of the hind legs, inability to stand, and finally, in severe cases, unconsciousness and death. Other symptoms sometimes noticed are rapid pulse, constipation or diarrhoea, partial blindness and abortion. Cattle develop similar, but milder, symptoms; the milk of poisoned cows has a bitter taste and the yield may drop. Poisoning in sheep is rare, but resembles that in cattle. Even when horsetail is no longer being eaten, poisoned animals take a long time to recover.

Veterinary attention should be sought as injections of vitamin B_1 may be needed.

● NOTE Care should be taken not to include horsetail when making hay.

ERICACEAE

This large family, consisting mainly of shrubs, includes low-growing woody plants such as heathers, large shrubs such as rhododendrons and azaleas, and a few trees. Some of the rhododendrons, notably *Rhododendron ponticum*, the species commonly found growing wild in Britain, are poisonous; the toxicity of the many individual cultivated species and varieties of rhododendron is not known. A few other garden plants in the family such as *Pieris* (see below) and others listed on page 99 produce a type of poisoning similar to that caused by rhododendron.

Pieris *Pieris formosa,Pieris japonica* and others (photo 31)

Various *Pieris* species are cultivated as ornamental shrubs in Britain. The mature leaves are up to 15 cm (6 in) long, about 2.5 cm (1 in) wide and are mid- or light-green; in some varieties the young leaves are a brilliant red. In autumn, small, usually white, bell-shaped flowers hang in a row of small clusters near the tip of the stems. There are many varieties, some with pink flowers and others with variegated leaves.

• POISONOUS SUBSTANCES These plants contain the same toxins as rhododendron, the most important one being acetylandromedol.

• POISONING No reports of human poisoning by *Pieris* have been found.

Most incidents have involved goats that have been allowed into gardens. Zoo animals have also been affected when they have browsed the shrub growing near their enclosures or after being fed the leaves by visitors. In general, the symptoms are similar to those of rhododendron poisoning, with vomiting, or attempts to vomit, being characteristic. Goats do not normally vomit, but they do so when poisoned by acetylandromedol. Other symptoms in goats are abdominal pain, grinding of teeth, shivering and blood-stained droppings. Material inhaled while vomiting can lead to pneumonia. Death of a foetus has been reported in a pregnant goat.

Veterinary care is required in these cases.

Rhododendron *Rhododendron ponticum* (photo 32)

Rhododendrons are not native in Britain, but since their introduction as garden shrubs, they have become naturalized in many places, often forming dense thickets and becoming dominant over other plants. Rhododendron is a branched, evergreen shrub, often with well developed trunk and branches. The leaves are tough and leathery, dark green above and paler beneath. They are elongated, smooth edged and pointed at each end. The large, cone-shaped buds develop into domed clusters of open, bell-shaped flowers, each up to 5 cm (2 in) across. Those of *Rhododendron ponticum*, the so-called 'wild' type, are a pale purple, but those of the many cultivated varieties have a wide range of colours. Azaleas, once treated as a separate genus, are now considered to

45

be rhododendrons. They are smaller shrubs with smaller flowers and have lighter-green leaves, and are not all evergreen,

- **POISONOUS SUBSTANCES** Various toxic diterpenoids have been identified, the most important being acetylandromedol, also known as andromedotoxin or grayanotoxin I. In those investigated, the whole plant contains the toxins, and these persist at least for a while after cutting. Rhododendrons vary in the amount of toxin they contain; in general, azaleas are of low toxicity.

- **POISONING** In this country it is most unlikely for circumstances to arise in which human poisoning could occur. In an unusual incident in Scotland, however, a man licked some drops of rhododendron nectar off his hand. In a very short time he experienced tingling in his fingers and toes, followed by numbness, loss of coordination and inability to stand. He had recovered completely a few hours later. Toxins present in rhododendron nectar can remain active in honey, and in countries where a considerable amount of the honey crop is derived from these plants, there can be similar symptoms, sometimes with vomiting and diarrhoea, if such honey is eaten. Only honey very recently produced by the bees is toxic, and this type of poisoning is most unlikely in Britain.

Many animals, but particularly cattle, sheep and goats, can be poisoned by rhododendrons. This can occur when fences are broken down, giving access to the bushes; in bad weather when other food is scarce; when the branches are weighed down by snow to within the reach of animals; and when garden refuse, with rhododendron trimmings, is thrown into fields. In all animals, the characteristic symptom of rhododendron poisoning is vomiting, even in animals that do not normally vomit. A greenish froth is often visible around the mouth and nose. Abdominal pain, constipation or diarrhoea, trembling, weakness and falling are also commonly observed; badly affected animals may die.

Purgatives are recommended for treatment.

- **NOTE** Great care should be taken not to let animals eat rhododendrons.

EUPHORBIACEAE

There are two groups of plants within this large family that grow wild in Britain, the spurges (*Euphorbia* species), and annual and dog's mercury (*Mercurialis* species). The milky or watery sap of these is known to be poisonous (see below); others, including the cultivated *Euphorbia* species and the house plants croton (*Codiaeum* species), have similar sap and can be poisonous, although the toxicity of many of the individual plants is not known. This family also includes the castor oil plant (*Ricinus communis*), which contains ricin one of the most potent plant toxins known (see below). For further details of other poisonous plants in the family see page 99.

Sun Spurge *Euphorbia helioscopia* (photo 34)

This rather striking, erect plant grows throughout Britain on cultivated or disturbed land such as field borders, gardens or roadsides. The plant grows up to 50 cm (20 in) tall and is smooth and bright or yellowish green. The stems may be single or branched, and bear small leaves, up to 2.5 cm (1 in) long, that are rounded at the tip and tapered towards the stem. When broken, the stems and leaves exude a white, milky sap that is characteristic of the spurges. Most of the plant is composed of the flowering stems, which divide into five 'rays' and then fork repeatedly near the top. At each fork there is a pair of leaf-like bracts that form cup-shaped structures within which are small, insignificant, yellowish-green flowers. For details of poisoning see under petty spurge below.

Petty Spurge *Euphorbia peplus* (photo 35)

Petty spurge is a common garden weed and also grows on waste ground throughout Britain. It is similar in general appearance to sun spurge but is smaller, 15–30 cm (6–12 in) high, with correspondingly smaller leaves and flowers. The flowering stems divide into three 'rays', and the paired bracts are oval or broadly triangular.

Of the many other spurges in Britain, the dwarf spurge (*Euphorbia exigua*) and the wood spurge (*Euphorbia amygdaloides*) are more likely to be seen than the rest, some of which have only a very restricted distribution in this country.

● POISONOUS SUBSTANCES The milky sap (latex) of these plants contains diterpene esters, which are not inactivated by drying.

● POISONING Children may be tempted to suck the 'milk' that exudes in drops from the cut stems of these plants. Even licking the fingers after handling the plant can produce symptoms. There is a strong, burning effect in the mouth and on the lips. Generally not enough is swallowed to produce severe symptoms, but, in Greece, two boys who sucked 'a quantity of ' the latex of sun spurge developed, in addition to burning of the mouth, severe stomach pain, vomiting, convulsions and coma. One boy died in four hours. The sap applied to the skin can cause a rash and blisters.

Spurges are not usually eaten by animals, but poisoning has been reported in horses, cattle and sheep with symptoms including excessive flow of saliva, inflammation and swelling of the mouth, and diarrhoea.

The skin and mouth should be rinsed thoroughly with warm water; if symptoms are severe, professional advice should be sought.

Poinsettia *Euphorbia pulcherrima* (photo 36)

This ornamental house plant is widely available, particularly at Christmas time. Most specimens grown in pots are 25–40 cm (10–16 in) high. The leaves are a dull green, pointed at the tip, sometimes uniformly oval in shape but usually having a few irregular indentations and pointed lobes. Small, uninteresting yellowish-red flowers develop in a compact group at the tips of the stems, but the 'leaves' immediately below them are the characteristic feature of the plant. Botanically these are not true leaves, but bracts, the name used specifically for the 'leaves' on a flower stalk. The bracts of poinsettia are almost as large as the leaves and a brilliant red, occasionally cream or white. The coloured bracts form a spectacular flat-topped crown to each stem.

• POISONOUS SUBSTANCES The milky sap of this plant contains various diterpene esters that are not destroyed by drying.

• POISONING The poinsettias commonly used as house plants appear to be much less toxic than they are often said to be, their reputation as dangerously poisonous plants apparently being based on a single report, in 1919, of a child in Hawaii dying after eating a few leaves; the reliability of this report has since been doubted. There may be differences in the toxicity of varieties, and in the susceptibility of individuals, and the plant should not be assumed to be completely non-toxic. In many human cases, mainly involving children who are attracted by the bright-red bracts, there are no symptoms at all, but in others there have been nausea, burning of the mouth and vomiting.

Poinsettia poisoning is rare in animals, but a fatal case has been recorded in a dog that ate a few poinsettia leaves after being left in a house on its own; it died in 12 hours after developing severe digestive-system disturbances.

It is unlikely that treatment would be required for human poisoning, but it is prudent to keep poinsettias out of the reach of pets.

Annual Mercury *Mercurialis annua*

Although widespread, particularly in southern England, annual mercury is not common. It is an annual plant that grows in waste places or as a garden weed, but is not necessarily found in the same place in successive years. The whole plant is smooth and bright green and the stems are erect, branched and of variable height, up to 50 cm (20 in), but often little more than 15 cm (6 in). The leaves are oval, stalked and usually less than 5 cm (2 in) long. The male and female flowers are borne on separate plants. For details of poisoning see under dog's mercury below.

Dog's Mercury *Mercurialis perennis* (photo 37)

This is a perennial plant, common in woods, where it spreads by underground stems into large areas, often to the exclusion of other plants. The plant is somewhat hairy and rough, with simple unbranched stems, 20–40 cm (8–16 in) tall. The dull-green, oval leaves are up to 7.5 cm (3 in) long, tapering towards the stalk and at the tip. They are present on the whole stem, but are closer together near the top. The male and female flowers grow on separate plants, the males in small clusters and the females singly or in pairs. When cut, the plant exudes a watery juice, particularly from the stems.

- POISONOUS SUBSTANCES Little is known about these, although methylamine (mercurialine), trimethylamine, a volatile oil and saponins are said to be present.
- POISONING Although there are some old reports of human poisoning by *Mercurialis*, this appears to be very rare, the only recent case being the result of mistaken identification. Dog's mercury, collected beside a stream, was boiled and eaten by two people who thought it was brooklime *(Veronica beccabunga)*. Nausea, vomiting and abdominal pains were experienced within three hours, together with sweating and flushing of the face. After hospital care, both recovered within 48 hours.

Animals do not often eat these plants, although some have been known to develop a liking for them. Poisoning has been reported in cattle, sheep, horses, pigs, goats and rabbits. Digestive-system disturbances, such as excessive production of saliva, signs of abdominal pain, constipation, then watery diarrhoea, develop first, followed by general weakness and painful urination; the urine is often reddish in colour and milk may be bluish. Occasionally the poisoning is fatal and coma may precede death.

Treatment, based on the replacement of lost body fluids, is required in all but very mild cases.

Castor Oil Plant *Ricinus communis* (photo 38)

This large annual plant is often planted in gardens, sometimes as a focal point in formal flower beds. The stalked leaves consist of usually eight radiating, pointed leaflets with slightly serrated edges and prominent central veins. Many varieties are green, but some are reddish brown. The flower spikes at the top of the stems are inconspicuous and often greenish (pink or red in the pigmented varieties), but the soft-spined fruits containing attractively mottled seeds are distinctive features of the plant. Although outside their normal climatic range, castor oil plants do sometimes produce seed in Britain.

- **POISONOUS SUBSTANCES** Ricin, a water-soluble simple protein, is present in the plant, with the highest concentration in the seeds; the toxicity remains even in dried seeds. Ricin is one of the most poisonous, naturally occurring substances known. Another protein that causes damage to red blood cells is also present, but is not toxic when taken by mouth; it is more readily destroyed by heating than ricin. Castor oil does not contain ricin.

- **POISONING** Human poisoning is most likely to result from eating the seeds (castor beans), although there are conflicting reports on the number of seeds that have caused severe or fatal poisoning. The ricin content and the size of the seeds may vary, and the amount of ricin released from them depends on how well they are chewed; a single seed has caused death, but people have recovered with suitable treatment, even after eating more than ten. Symptoms begin within a few hours with abdominal pain, vomiting and diarrhoea (sometimes with blood) that may last for several days, causing severe dehydration. There is decreased production of urine and a fall in blood pressure. If death has not occurred in three to five days, the patient usually recovers. Wearing or playing with necklaces made of castor beans should be avoided, as swelling and soreness of the skin may result. Babies who chew such necklaces can be severely poisoned.

In 1978, ricin was thought to have been used for the assassination of Georgi Markov, a Bulgarian journalist living in Britain. A perforated metallic pellet, presumed to have contained the toxin, was found embedded in his leg after he had been jabbed with an umbrella while waiting at a bus stop near Waterloo Station in London.

Castor beans, after being crushed to remove the oil, are used as an ingredient of animal feeds. If properly prepared, such feed is harmless, but poisoning has occurred in cattle and pigs when the necessary heat treatment has been inadequate and the ricin not completely destroyed. The most prominent symptoms are abdominal pain and diarrhoea, often with blood; severe vomiting occurs in pigs. Horses and poultry have been poisoned by the accidental incorporation of castor beans into their food. In an isolated instance, dogs died after eating a 'biological' fertilizer containing castor beans.

Professional treatment is essential as castor bean poisoning is potentially fatal in both man and animals.

- **NOTE** This plant is dangerously poisonous; it contains one of the most potent toxins known.

FAGACEAE

Oaks (*Quercus* species) and particularly their acorns are an important source of poisoning in farm animals. Little is known about variations in the toxicity of individual species. Poisoning has also been caused by beech (*Fagus sylvatica*).

Beech *Fagus sylvatica* (photo 39)

Beech is a large, much branched tree, up to 40 m (130 ft) high, that grows mainly on chalky soils in the southern parts of the country. In some places, whole areas of woodland are almost exclusively beech. Ornamental varieties, such as copper beech, are also grown; both types are used for hedges. The trunk and branches have a smooth, grey bark, the leaf buds are brown, slender and pointed, and the leaves oval, 5–10 cm (2–4 in) long; they are a delicate light green in spring, but darken later. In autumn, brown, spiny or scaly husks fall to the ground, often in very large numbers; they contain triangular seeds (beech nuts), each about 1 cm (⅓ in) long, and covered in a thin, brown skin that becomes brittle when ripe.

• POISONOUS SUBSTANCES Little is known about the toxic constituents of beech, but a substance called fagin, the chemical composition of which is not clearly defined, is said to be present, particularly in the husks surrounding the seeds.

• POISONING It is only the seeds (nuts) of beech that are likely to cause human poisoning. If only a few are eaten, symptoms are limited to soreness of the mouth and throat, but larger quantities (50 or more) have produced headache, digestive-system disturbances (stomach ache, vomiting, diarrhoea), dizziness and an increase in body temperature; there may also be weakness and fainting. These symptoms appear about an hour after eating beech nuts and may persist for several hours.

It used to be a common practice to crush beech nuts with their surrounding husk to extract the oil, the residue being used in animal feed; this sometimes gave rise to poisoning, particularly in horses and cattle. It is also dangerous to feed whole beech nuts to animals; fatal poisoning has been reported in horses that ate 300–500 g (10–18 oz). The symptoms are similar to, but more severe than, those of human poisoning; there may be violent abdominal pain, staggering, paralysis and unconsciousness.

Professional advice should be sought in cases of severe poisoning.

Oak *Quercus* species (photo 40)

There are two common oaks in Britain, the pedunculate oak (*Quercus robur*) and the sessile oak (*Quercus petraea*); several foreign species are also planted in parks and gardens. Oaks are large, usually deciduous, trees up to 30 m (100 ft) tall, with rough, fissured bark and broad, spreading branches; some trees live for many hundreds of years. The British oaks have dull-green leaves (shiny, bright green and often tinged red when young) up to 10 cm (4 in) long. They have characteristic, smoothly indented wavy margins; other oaks have leaves with pointed lobes. Male catkins and small, inconspicuous female flowers develop on the same tree in spring. The smooth, oval seeds (acorns) are about 2.5 cm (1 in) long, each partially enclosed in a woody cup with an irregular surface covered with small raised dots or stiff hairs, according to the species. When ripe, the acorns become brown and fall from the trees, often still within their cups.

● POISONOUS SUBSTANCES Tannins occur in all parts of the tree, but particularly in young leaves and green acorns; extracts from the bark were used for tanning leather. There have been suggestions that other toxic substances, including those produced by fungi, may also be present.

● POISONING Children may occasionally eat a few acorns, but this is no cause for alarm.

In animals, serious poisoning may result from eating large quantities of oak leaves or acorns. Cattle are most commonly affected, but oak poisoning has also been reported in horses, sheep, deer and (rarely) pigs. The most likely time for this to happen is in early autumn. After the long, hot summer of 1984, when the acorn crop was very heavy and good grazing was scarce, there was an unusually high incidence of acorn poisoning in cattle in Britain. It may be a few days before the symptoms appear, but sometimes, as in 1984, some animals die suddenly. The milk of poisoned cows has a bitter taste. The digestive system is affected, initially with loss of appetite, abdominal distension and pain, and constipation often associated with groaning and considerable straining. Later there is dark-coloured diarrhoea with blood. Severely affected animals have kidney damage, which is sometimes fatal. Particularly in horses there may also be foaming around the mouth, loss of coordination, and convulsions. In the past, when acorns were collected for feeding pigs, they caused poisoning only if excessive quantities were eaten; when given as only part of the feed, acorns ground into meal have been used safely.

Individual animals may develop a craving for acorns and oak leaves. Even before recovering from the effects of poisoning, they may try to return to oak trees, sometimes breaking down fences in the process. The craving may persist in subsequent years.

Veterinary advice should be sought in cases of poisoning by the leaves or acorns of oak.

HIPPOCASTANACEAE

In this family, the large horse chestnut and buckeye trees (*Aesculus* species) are poisonous. Their seeds, 'conkers', are responsible for most of the cases of poisoning.

Horse Chestnut *Aesculus hippocastanum* (photo 41)

This large deciduous tree, up to 30 m (100 ft) tall, is often planted, sometimes in rows or avenues, in parks, streets and large gardens. In spring the thick twigs bear large buds covered with sticky, brown scales. These buds develop into large, coarse, stalked leaves, with five to seven, elongated, radiating leaflets that are broader and rounded towards the tip. Before the leaves have expanded, the new shoots are densely covered with hairs. In late spring, spikes of creamy-white flowers, sometimes red or pink, grow at the tips of the branches. In autumn, tough, green fruits with a few coarse spines form; these contain the characteristic, large seeds, or conkers, that have a dull, pale patch on one side but are otherwise a grained, glossy reddish brown.

● POISONOUS SUBSTANCE A saponic glycoside, called aesculin after the Latin name of the tree, is present, particularly in the bark, flowers and young leaves, but the seeds (conkers) are also poisonous.

● POISONING Despite their bitter taste, children sometimes eat conkers, but seldom in sufficient quantities to cause severe poisoning; a mild stomach upset, with vomiting, is all that usually results. Eating large numbers, however, can be serious, leading to unconsciousness and even death; such incidents are extremely rare.

In parkland, the leaves of horse chestnut trees are browsed by animals with no apparent ill effect, although poisoning, most probably by the conkers, has been reported in cattle, horses and pigs. Symptoms include inflammation of the digestive system, weakness, uncoordinated movement, paralysis and coma.

Severe poisoning requires professional care.

HYPERICACEAE

This family contains many plants, including several shrubs, grown in gardens in Britain, but it is the wild species, particularly perforate St. John's wort (*Hypericum perforatum*, see below) that can be harmful, as they sometimes grow on land grazed by farm animals.

Perforate St. John's Wort *Hypericum perforatum* (photo 42)

This perennial plant grows wild throughout most of the country in hedgerows, rough grassland, open woodland and on road verges, and is the most common St. John's wort in Britain; others have only limited distribution. Several garden species and varieties are also grown. Smooth, erect, two-ridged stems, 30 cm–1 m (1-3 ft) tall, grow up in spring from the woody base of the plant and bear paired leaves. These have no stalks and are less than 2.5 cm (1 in) long; they are narrow where they join the stem, then widen slightly before tapering towards the rounded or slightly pointed tip. On the leaves are numerous small black dots that appear translucent when viewed against the light. These are a characteristic feature of some, but not all, *Hypericum* species. Several clusters of flowers, each 1–2 cm (⅓–¾ in) across, develop near the top of the stem. The five radiating petals and the numerous stamens in the centre of the flower are bright yellow.

● POISONOUS SUBSTANCE A pigment, called hypericin, which sensitizes the skin to sunlight, is present in the small black dots on the leaves. The reaction, called photosensitization, can still develop after eating the dried plant (for example, when mixed in hay), although much of the pigment will have been destroyed.

● POISONING People are unlikely to eat this plant and no cases of human poisoning have been reported.

Poisoning in animals affects only those having unpigmented areas of skin with little hair; dark-skinned animals are not affected. When susceptible animals are exposed to strong sunlight after eating the plant, the unpigmented areas of their body, especially around the eyes and muzzle, become red and swollen, with fluid exuding and drying to form scabs. There is also irritation of the affected areas which causes the animals to become restless and rub against trees and fences; in severe cases even deep layers of skin can be lost. More severe symptoms occur in horses than in cattle, sheep or pigs.

The most important aspect of treatment is to remove the animals from direct sunlight, preferably by housing them, after which they should recover in a few days.

IRIDACEAE

Although the toxicity of the individual species and varieties of iris is not known, both wild and cultivated plants have caused poisoning in animals. Gladioli, also members of this family, can cause mild poisoning (see page 100).

Iris *Iris* species (photo 43)

The two irises that grow wild in Britain are the yellow flag (*Iris pseudacorus*), which is found at the edges of ponds and rivers and in swampy ground, and the pale-purple flowered stinking iris or gladdon (*Iris foetidissima*) that grows, usually on chalky soil, in open woods or hedgerows and on cliffs near the sea. Many species and varieties are grown in gardens. Most have a thick, fleshy underground stem (rhizome) with prominent ridges round it, where buds develop to form the leaves. These are up to 1 m (3 ft) long in some cultivated plants, but smaller in the wild species; they are pointed and flat except near the base, where they arise opposite each other, with overlapping sheaths. The leaves of many irises are a pale, slightly bluish green, but others are darker. The flowers are of various colours and have a characteristic shape, with upper segments erect but tending to arch over the broad lower lobes, which turn downwards, revealing the inner part of the flower. These lower lobes are usually distinctively marked, often in different or darker colours.

● POISONOUS SUBSTANCE This is thought to be a glycoside, called iridin or irisin. All parts of the plant are poisonous, and remain so even after drying.

● POISONING Severe vomiting and diarrhoea, sometimes with bleeding, have been reported on the rare occasions when people have eaten parts of *Iris* plants. The sap from irises can irritate the skin and cause blistering.

Poisoning is more likely to occur in animals that may eat wild or garden irises or hay containing the dried plants. The effects are similar to those of human poisoning and have been described in cattle, horses and pigs. In one instance, some calves died after eating irises from a garden border. Pigs also died when they ate the rhizomes exposed during dredging.

● NOTE Care should be taken in disposing of rhizomes, as animals may be particularly attracted to fleshy parts of plants left on the surface of the ground.

LEGUMINOSAE

This large family, sometimes called Papilionaceae, contains many well-known food plants, such as peas and beans, and also important fodder crops, such as clover, for animals. Under some circumstances, however, these may cause poisoning (see Crop plants, page 91). The garden tree, laburnum *(Laburnum anagyroides)*, and lupins *(Lupinus* species*)* have poisoned both children and animals (see below). Other plants in this family that may cause poisoning are listed on page 101.

Laburnum *Laburnum anagyroides* (photos 44 and 45)
Golden Rain; Golden Chain

This small tree is common in parks and gardens, but is occasionally seen growing in a semi-wild state. The trunk is usually less than 20 cm (8 in) in diameter and has dark, fairly smooth, brownish-green bark. When the leaves develop in spring, they are downy and folded at first, then open out into usually three oval leaflets on a slender stalk. The flowers form characteristic, long, delicate, hanging clusters, each flower being bright yellow and about 2 cm (¾ in) across. Bunches of green seed pods form after flowering; they dry and become brown in autumn, then split open to shed the seeds. Some cultivated laburnums do not set seed and rarely form pods.

● POISONOUS SUBSTANCE An alkaloid, cytisine, is present in the whole tree, but particularly in the bark and seeds. Apparently the toxicity of the leaves decreases, while that of the flowers and fruits increases as they develop.

● POISONING This is the plant most frequently suspected of causing human poisoning in this country. In the past, there have been reports of very serious and even fatal poisoning which are frequently quoted; these can give rise to great alarm and anxiety. Although these reports tend to exaggerate the dangers of laburnum, it is none the less advisable to keep suspected cases under close observation. Children are the most likely to be poisoned by laburnum, when they eat the small green pods or the seeds within them; chewing the flowers can also cause poisoning. Symptoms usually develop within an hour and include burning of the mouth and throat, stomach ache, diarrhoea, and persistent vomiting, followed by drowsiness, dizziness, headache, difficult breathing and dilated pupils. In many cases the spontaneous vomiting eliminates the toxins and recovery is complete after 24 hours.

There are isolated reports of laburnum poisoning in most domestic animals, but in general such poisoning is rare. Horses and cattle have shown muscular tremors, loss of coordination, abdominal pain and coma; some have died. A pig that ate laburnum leaves with lawn mowings developed profuse diarrhoea. Dogs have been poisoned by chewing laburnum; one died in convulsions within half an hour.

Because of the possibility of serious symptoms developing, professional advice should be sought.

Lupin *Lupinus* species (photo 46)

The lupins found in this country are varieties of *Lupinus polyphyllus*; they are garden plants but occasionally become naturalized and persist for a few years in a semi-wild state. The best known are Russell lupins, named after the man who developed them. The plants grow as clumps of leaves, with 12–18 slender, pointed leaflets, up to 12.5 cm (5 in) long, radiating from the top of the stalk. Spikes of densely packed flowers, up to 1.5 m (5 ft) tall, grow in summer. The original 'wild-type' lupin had bluish-purple flowers, but now varieties are available in a wide range of colours. After flowering the seed pods develop; they are green and velvety at first, then dry to a greyish brown and split open to reveal a row of dark-brown seeds.

The tree lupin *(Lupinus arboreus)* is also grown here. It is a semi-woody shrub 1.5–2.5 m (5–8 ft) high and a similar width. The leaves are the same as those of the Russell lupins, but somewhat smaller, and the flowers are yellow, occasionally white.

Attempts are being made to grow here the lupins used abroad for animal feed, but so far this has not been particularly successful.

● POISONOUS SUBSTANCES Various alkaloids are present in lupins, the seeds in particular containing high concentrations. Drying and storage do not eliminate the toxicity. There are, however, some varieties that contain only insignificant amounts of toxic alkaloids.

● POISONING Human poisoning is likely to occur only if children eat the small green pods or chew the seeds contained in the attractive, velvety pods. Eating two or more pods or their seeds can cause nausea, vomiting, abdominal pain, headache and dizziness.

Lupin poisoning in animals in this country could occur if they gain access to gardens, or if garden refuse is thrown onto their pasture. In countries where lupins are grown as a fodder crop, the alkaloids can cause restlessness, staggering and convulsions in older and deformity in newborn animals. This problem is decreasing as new varieties of so-called sweet lupins, with low alkaloid content, are being introduced. Another disease, known as lupinosis, has occurred in several countries after animals have eaten lupins infected with fungi; the symptoms are slower to develop and result from liver damage.

LILIACEAE

Some members of this large family present in Britain are poisonous. These include wild plants, such as bog asphodel *(Narthecium ossifragum)* and bluebell *(Hyacinthoides non-scripta)* and several house and garden plants. The most important are described below, and others are listed on page 102.

Autumn Crocus *Colchicum autumnale* (photo 47)
Meadow Saffron; Naked Ladies

Autumn crocuses are seen far more often as garden plants than growing wild, although in a few localities they are still plentiful, usually in damp meadows and woods. The flowers are the most noticeable feature of these plants as they develop in autumn, after the leaves have died down, and are the only parts of the plant clearly visible at that stage. The basal part of the flower is a slender whitish tube, 5–15 cm (2–6 in) high, arising at ground level. This widens into the upper part of the flower that has usually six pink or purple petal-like lobes, superficially resembling spring crocuses. The flowers are delicate and easily flattened by wind or rain. After flowering, an oval fruit forms at the base of the flower tube, where it remains until spring, when the flower stalk grows, raising the elongated, oval fruits well above ground level among the leaves that develop at the same time. The leaves are shiny and bright green, with prominent parallel veins. They often exceed 20 cm (8 in) in length and are narrow at the base but tend to widen higher up, to about 4 cm (1½ in) before tapering to a point at the tip.

• POISONOUS SUBSTANCES Alkaloids (colchicine and colchiceine) are present in all parts of the plant, but especially the corm and the seeds. The dried plant is still toxic.

• POISONING Children have been poisoned by eating flowers and also leaves, but it is the seeds that are more likely to attract their attention, as, when ripe, they rattle if the seed head is shaken. Human poisoning can also occur if the corms are mistaken for onions, or by drinking milk from cows that have eaten the plant. There may be a delay of several hours before the appearance of symptoms; these include burning of the mouth and throat, difficulty in swallowing, abdominal pain, nausea, vomiting and diarrhoea, sometimes with blood. In severe cases, poisoning may lead to collapse, convulsions, paralysis and death. Such poisoning is, however, rare, as people are not likely to eat sufficient quantities of the plant.

Similar symptoms, sometimes with a fatal outcome, have occurred in cattle, sheep, horses, pigs and goats.

If poisoning is suspected, treatment should be started even before symptoms appear; professional advice is needed.

Lily of the Valley *Convallaria majalis* (photo 48)

In the past, this shade-loving spring plant grew wild in many parts of the country, particularly in eastern areas. It is now less widespread, but is commonly grown in gardens and wooded parks. A pair of broad, elliptical leaves, pointed at the tip, grow from a creeping underground stem, and from between them the flower stalk, rarely exceeding 15 cm (6 in) in height, develops. It bears, on one side, 6–12 small, white, bell-shaped flowers, noted for their fragrance. As the flowers wither in late spring, spherical, green berries can be seen; these become soft and red when ripe.

• POISONOUS SUBSTANCES Lily of the valley contains several glycosides including convallotoxin, convalloside, and convallamarin and also saponins. The whole plant is poisonous, but most cases of poisoning arise after the berries have been eaten.

• POISONING Some of the most frequent plant poisoning queries received by

Poison Information Centres relate to this plant, and usually involve children who have eaten the attractive red berries. The symptoms of poisoning include nausea, vomiting and abdominal pain; headache, dilated pupils, mental disturbance and irregular or slow heart beat have been reported and, in extreme cases, coma and death from heart failure. Serious poisoning is rare, however, as vomiting limits the absorption of the toxins.

Although sometimes said to be dangerously poisonous to livestock, there is little evidence to support this. Lily of the valley should, however, be considered as potentially poisonous to animals because of its constituents.

If there are more than mild symptoms, professional advice should be sought.

• NOTE The ability of the plant to induce vomiting and affect heart beat led, in former times, to its being used medicinally.

Bluebell *Hyacinthoides non-scripta* (photo 49)
Wild Hyacinth

Bluebells are common throughout Britain, mainly in woodland, where they may cover large areas of ground and appear as a blue 'carpet' when flowering in spring. The plant grows from white bulbs beneath the ground. Narrow, bright-green leaves, up to 30 cm (12 in) long, develop first, followed by smooth, round flower stalks that bear blue, bell-shaped flowers about 1 cm (⅓ in) long. These are grouped close together and hang down near the top of the stalk. Oval fruits up to 1.5 cm (½ in) across develop in late spring. They are green at first, but become light brown and dry as the seeds mature.

• POISONOUS SUBSTANCES The whole plant contains glycosides, named scillarens after a former name of the plant *(Scilla)*. These affect the heart in a similar way to the glycosides of foxgloves.

• POISONING Human poisoning has occurred when bluebell bulbs have been mistaken for onions. Abdominal pain, diarrhoea, and slow, weak pulse have resulted. Diarrhoea was reported in a young child who ate six to ten seed pods of bluebells after flowering. The sap of bluebells and related plants, such as hyacinths and *Ornithogalum* species, can cause dermatitis.

There have been sporadic reports of bluebell poisoning in animals; a horse was poisoned by the bulbs, and cattle by the foliage. Initially there are digestive-system disturbances and, later, effects on the heart, including a slow, weak, erratic pulse.

Bog Asphodel *Narthecium ossifragum* (photo 50)

This small plant grows, often in considerable numbers, on wet heaths, bogs and moorland throughout Britain, but more commonly in the west and north. The whole plant is stiff and erect, except the tips of the uniformly narrow, flattish leaves, that tend to curve downwards. The leaves are 5–30 cm (2–12 in) long and are flattened into a sheath at ground level. The flowers develop in summer on a single stalk that has a few small, clasping leaves (bracts). Near the top of the stalk is a spike of small, bright-yellow flowers, each about 1 cm (⅓ in) across, and consisting of several narrow, petal-like structures surrounding the central, orange stamens. After flowering, every part of the flower stalk becomes dark orange and is thus still clearly visible among the surrounding vegetation.

● **POISONOUS SUBSTANCES** Saponins, particularly narthecin, are present. The highest concentrations are in the flowers and the tips of the leaves.

● **POISONING** There are no reports of human poisoning.

In animals, poisoning has been reported only in sheep and lambs, and was first described in Norway, under the name 'alveld' (elf fire). This appears to be the same as diseases called 'plochteach', 'yellowses' and 'head greet' in Scotland, 'saut' in Cumbria, and 'heddles' or 'hard lug' in Co. Antrim. The connection between these conditions and bog asphodel in Britain has been recognized only comparatively recently. The saponins cause liver damage, which leads to the accumulation in the blood of a substance (phylloerythrin) that makes the skin of the sheep sensitive to sunlight (photosensitization). The areas chiefly affected are those with unpigmented skin and little or no wool, such as the face, ears and feet. They become red, hot and swollen; fluid exudes and dries to form hard crusts and the skin may be broken. In severe cases, the tips of the ears may be lost, and some animals become blind. The liver damage may result in death, even in black animals whose skin is unaffected. Sheep do not generally eat bog asphodel if there is plenty of good grass available.

Affected sheep should be removed from areas where bog asphodel is plentiful; shading from the sun is desirable. Veterinary help should be sought if the symptoms are severe.

Solomon's Seal *Polygonatum multiflorum* (photo 51)

This is usually considered a garden plant, although in a few localities it grows wild or may be found semi-wild as a garden escape. There are several cultivated varieties and hybrids. Solomon's seal has underground stems, from which graceful, arching stems, up to 60 cm (2 ft) long develop in spring. These bear elongated, pointed leaves, arising horizontally on either side of the stem, and clusters of two to five small, tubular, green-edged, white flowers that hang down from the point of attachment of the leaves. Blue or black berries develop in late spring and can persist until autumn.

● **POISONOUS SUBSTANCES** The plant is said to contain saponins, but there is very little known about them, except that their concentration is particularly high in the seeds.

● POISONING Solomon's seal berries have caused poisoning in children who have eaten them, but no details are available.

In animals a case of poisoning recently reported in Britain involved a puppy, which ate some leaves of the plant and developed vomiting that persisted for several days.

False Hellebore *Veratrum* species (photo 52)
False Helleborine; White Hellebore

These plants should not be confused with the true hellebores *(Helleborus* species), which belong to the Ranunculaceae family.

False hellebores are not found wild in Britain, but are sometimes planted in gardens, usually in shady places. They grow from underground stems and the flower stalks are up to 1.5 m (5 ft) high. The leaves, often 30 cm (12 in) long, have parallel veins, the leaf surface being ridged between them. The leaves grow close together, sheathing each other near the base. Large numbers of closely packed, star-like, usually greenish- or yellowish-white flowers, sometimes red, depending on the variety, develop on the tall flower spike in midsummer. The small seed pods that form after flowering turn black as they ripen.

● POISONOUS SUBSTANCES There are steroidal alkaloids in all parts of these plants, but especially in the rootstock and leaves.

● POISONING It is unlikely that people will eat false hellebores, but they can cause serious poisoning, with burning in the mouth and throat, abdominal pain, vomiting, diarrhoea, and muscular twitching and cramp. In severe cases the heart is affected, giving a slow, weak pulse; there may also be difficulty in breathing, coldness, trembling, collapse and death.

False hellebores have also poisoned cattle, sheep and goats, which have shown symptoms similar to those described for human poisoning. Animals that eat false hellebores during pregnancy often have severely deformed young.

Professional advice should be sought urgently if *Veratrum* poisoning is suspected.

LORANTHACEAE

The only member of this family likely to be found in Britain is *Viscum album* (see below). Other mistletoes such as *Loranthus* species and the American *Phoradrendron* are also poisonous.

Mistletoe *Viscum album* (photo 53)

Mistletoe is a partial parasite, having green leaves, but always growing on trees, where it forms a characteristic, bushy mass, often more or less spherical and usually 60 cm (2 ft) or less across. It grows on many types of tree, but rarely on evergreens or conifers. The stems are green, tough and branching, with smooth, leathery leaves, often about 5 cm (2 in) long and 1–2 cm (⅓–¾ in) across. Compact groups of inconspicuous greenish-yellow flowers grow in spring and develop in autumn into waxy, white, slightly translucent berries that contain a thick, somewhat sticky juice and a single seed. These often remain throughout the winter.

● POISONOUS SUBSTANCES Mistletoe contains toxic proteins, named viscotoxins A and B; the leaves and stems are said to be more poisonous than the berries. The toxicity of the plant varies according to the tree on which it is growing; for example, mistletoe on lime or poplar trees is more poisonous than that on apple trees.

● POISONING Queries about human poisoning are most likely to arise when mistletoe is cut and brought indoors at Christmas time. Children sometimes eat the berries, but poisoning is rarely serious. The severity of the reaction depends on the number of berries eaten; a few berries may have no effect at all or cause only mild stomach ache, whereas eating the leaves or a large number of berries may lead to more serious digestive disturbances, including stomach cramps and diarrhoea, sometimes with blood. It should be emphasized that reactions to eating mistletoe are very variable and even fatal poisoning has been recorded.

Pets are also at risk at Christmas; dogs have been poisoned, some fatally, by eating mistletoe. They become agitated, uncoordinated and sensitive to touch, particularly on the abdomen. Similar symptoms have been reported in a horse.

For treatment it is recommended that vomiting should be induced.

OLEACEAE

The only members of this family known to have caused poisoning in Britain are the ash tree *(Fraxinus excelsior)* and privet *(Ligustrum* species). Other species and varieties of both are cultivated here, but it is not known how their toxicity differs from that of the native species.

Ash *Fraxinus excelsior* (photo 54)

Ash trees are common in parks, woods, scrub and hedges throughout most of Britain, although less so on acid soils. When left untrimmed, they grow as stately trees up to 24 m (80 ft) high, with spreading branches and smooth, grey bark, cracked on older parts. The twigs and small branches tend to snap readily; they bear roughly triangular buds, up to 1 cm (⅓ in) across, which have a sooty appearance. The leaves are on long stalks and consist of a terminal leaflet and up to 12 paired lateral leaflets, all of which are a similar size, up to 4 cm (1½ in) long, and oval, with a pointed tip. The small flowers form before the leaves and have a purplish appearance (the colour of the stamens); these develop into the characteristic bunches of 'keys', the winged seeds that hang from the trees in autumn and sometimes persist through the winter.

- POISONOUS SUBSTANCES Little is known about these, but ash is said to contain glycosides, including aesculin, the main toxic agent in horse chestnut (*Aesculus hippocastanum*).

- POISONING No reports of human poisoning have been found.

The information on the toxicity of ash for animals is somewhat contradictory. In some parts of the country, such as the Lake District, it is customary to cut branches from ash trees and give them to cattle, whereas poisoning of cattle by ash is well recognized in other parts, such as the Midlands, where it is called 'wood evil'. This condition arises from eating leaves and fruits, particularly in autumn, when large quantities often fall to the ground (still green) after a sharp frost. The stomach (rumen) becomes filled with a solid mass of leaves; rumination ceases, and there is constipation, with grunting sounds and signs of abdominal pain. Two cows that ate leaves and fruits from a fallen branch also became drowsy and uncoordinated. It has been suggested that fungi growing on the foliage during wet autumn weather are responsible for some of the toxicity of ash. This and the variable amounts eaten could account for the conflicting reports on its toxicity, but at present there is no conclusive evidence.

Veterinary advice should be sought as it may be necessary to remove the stomach contents.

Privet *Ligustrum* species (photo 55)

Wild privet (*Ligustrum vulgare*) is a branched shrub native to southern Britain, where it is found particularly on chalky soils. Garden privet (*Ligustrum ovalifolium*), introduced from Japan, has become a very popular hedge plant. The wild species has narrow, pointed, smooth leaves that are bright green and shiny when young, but become darker and dull as they mature; those of the cultivated garden privet are shorter, rarely more than 3 cm (1¼ in) long and are more oval in shape, and in some varieties may be yellow or variegated. Small, white flowers with a tubular base, expanded near the opening, form in vertical, roughly cone-shaped clusters in summer; they have a characteristic, sweetish smell. Groups of small, shiny, black berries appear in autumn.

● **POISONOUS SUBSTANCE** The nature of this is not known precisely, but it is usually stated to be the glycoside ligustrin. It is present in the whole plant, but the berries are particularly poisonous.

● **POISONING** Eating a small number of privet berries can cause vomiting, abdominal pain and diarrhoea. Fatal poisoning by privet is rare, but recently in Germany a two-year-old boy died within three hours of eating privet berries from a hedge around a playground, and two of four slightly older children died in similar circumstances in Russia; the number of berries they had eaten was not known. The children had convulsions and an irregular heart beat before death.

Poisoning is rare in animals, but can be severe or even fatal. The most likely source is hedge trimmings thrown onto pasture. Horses have died within 48 hours of eating privet, and, in one case, only four hours after browsing an overgrown hedge. Initially there is staggering and abdominal pain and later, paralysis. Cattle and sheep have also been poisoned.

Because of the potentially dangerous nature of privet poisoning, professional advice should be sought.

PAPAVERACEAE

Various wild and cultivated poppies found in Britain are poisonous (see below and page 104). The family also contains greater celandine (*Chelidonium majus*) used for centuries as a medicinal plant; it can be poisonous.

Greater Celandine *Chelidonium majus* (photo 56)

Greater celandine grows in banks and hedgerows, often near buildings. Its frequent association with old buildings is probably linked with its former medicinal uses. It is a perennial plant that is branched and woody near the base, on which some leaves persist throughout the winter. Each year flowering stems, 30–60 cm (1–2 ft) tall, develop, with oval or pointed, slightly bluish-green leaves that have a wavy margin and widen at the base of the stalk where they join the stem; the upper leaves may have three distinct lobes. The flowers are up to 2 cm (¾ in) across, and have four, rounded, yellow petals. The seed capsules are rather like small pods, very narrow in diameter and up to 5 cm (2 in) long.

● **POISONOUS SUBSTANCES** The whole plant contains a mixture of alkaloids, including chelidonine and chelerythrine. Their toxic activity is greatly reduced in dried plants.

• POISONING In the past, medicinal preparations of the plant produced a variety of undesirable side effects, but there are no recent reports of human poisoning. The death of a four-year-old boy in 1936 was attributed to greater celandine, and the reputation of this plant as a cause of fatal poisoning seems to be based on this one incident. The sap of the plant is reputed to cause blistering of the skin, although one or two experiments have cast doubt on this.

The plant has an acrid taste and an unpleasant smell and is rarely eaten by animals. Poisoning did occur in cattle, however, when they ate greater celandine at the seeding stage; they had been unaffected by eating it earlier in the season. The animals showed an increased flow of saliva, thirst, drowsiness and staggering. There were violent convulsions when the animals were touched. Other reports mention severe diarrhoea.

Field Poppy *Papaver rhoeas* (photo 57)
Common Poppy; Corn Poppy

This delicate annual plant, once very common in corn fields, was almost eliminated from some areas by weed-killers, but is now increasing again. It is often seen on banks and road verges; several varieties are grown in gardens. The plant grows up to 60 cm (2 ft) tall. The leaves are deeply indented and toothed, and they and the flowering stem are covered with bristly hairs. The oval flower buds hang down from the top of the stalk, but become erect as the bright-red flowers open. These are 5–10 cm (2–4 in) across and have four rounded petals, each with a large dark blotch at the base, where there is a mass of bluish-green or blackish stamens. The seed heads (capsules) are rounded at the base, but flat at the top, where there are radiating dark lines. The seeds are very numerous, and when ripe and dry can be shaken from the capsule through small holes that develop just below the flat disc.

• POISONOUS SUBSTANCES Various alkaloids are present in all parts of the plants.

• POISONING The field poppy and its garden varieties are unlikely to cause human poisoning.

It is only when poppies are eaten in fairly large quantities that they will cause poisoning in animals. This has occurred when garden poppies have been discarded and thrown on to pasture. Horses, cattle and sheep have become restless and uncoordinated and developed muscular twitching and stiffness. They may fall and be unable to rise; in some cases the abdomen is bloated. Although such poisoning is rarely fatal, it may take many months for animals to recover. The yield of milking cows may remain low.

Opium Poppy *Papaver somniferum*

This annual plant is not a British species, but grows in many places throughout the country and is often cultivated in gardens. The leaves are greyish green and have irregularly wavy or toothed edges. The flowering stems are smooth or sparsely hairy and grow up to 45 cm (18 in tall), and the leaves (bracts) on them clasp the stem. The large flowers may be up to 15 cm (6 in) across, but are usually slightly smaller. The four pale, pinkish-purple or whitish petals (crinkled in some varieties) are curved slightly upwards to form a shallow cup. In some varieties there is a dark blotch at the base of each petal. The stamens are greyish and very numerous; they form a ring round the central capsule. This is a bluish green, more or less spherical structure, with a flat disc on the top that has radiating dark lines on its surface, and a regularly wavy edge. The tiny blackish seeds are shed through small holes that develop just below the disc as the seed head dries.

• POISONOUS SUBSTANCES Various alkaloids are present, mainly in the milky sap (latex) of the seed capsule, but also in other parts of the plant, except the seeds, which can be used safely. The drug opium is prepared by drying the latex.

• POISONING The dangers involved in the misuse of the prepared drug, opium, are well known, but simple extracts of the plant can also be dangerous; a fatal human case has been reported in which opium poppy seed capsules were boiled in water and drunk as tea.

Poisoning has occurred in cattle fed stalks and seed capsules. The symptoms included extreme restlessness, constant lowing, excessive flow of saliva, digestive-system disturbances, decreased body temperature, increased rate of breathing and finally, deep sleep. Recovery is slow, and the milk yield of cows remains low. Poisoning has also been reported in two dogs that ate opium poppies growing in a garden.

Professional advice should be sought urgently in cases of suspected poisoning by opium poppies and preparations made from them.

• NOTE The poppy seeds used by bakers for decorating bread are harmless.

PHYTOLACCACEAE

This family is not native to Britain, but one introduced species, *Phytolacca americana*, is not uncommon and can cause poisoning.

Pokeweed *Phytolacca americana*
Inkweed; Pokeberry

This American plant is grown in Britain in gardens, but occasionally becomes established elsewhere and grows in a semi-wild state. It is a coarse, unpleasant-smelling perennial with branched succulent stems up to 3 m (10 ft) tall, although in the British climate it rarely reaches this height. The leaves have elongated, oval leaflets, which are pointed at the tip and have prominent veins. The tiny greenish-white flowers, pinkish in some cultivated varieties, are densely crowded to form erect spikes. Purplish-black fruits with staining, reddish juice develop in autumn.

● POISONOUS SUBSTANCES There is little definite information about these, but triterpenoid saponins, including phytolaccin and phytolaccatoxin, are present. The root is the most toxic, but the toxicity of the whole plant increases as it grows; the unripe berries and seeds are also particularly poisonous. The ripe berries are the least poisonous; in the USA they are cooked in pies, but when eaten raw they can cause poisoning.

● POISONING If berries develop on garden specimens, children sometimes eat them and, after a delay of an hour or two, they may have stomach cramps, vomiting and diarrhoea. A few berries may be harmless for older children and adults, but cause serious poisoning in small children. With larger quantities, the digestive-system symptoms can be severe, and drowsiness, coma and even death may occur. A man who ate the roots of pokeweek, having mistaken them for horse radish, experienced soreness of the mouth, severe, persistent vomiting, dizziness, and difficulty in breathing; he took 48 hours to recover. The sap from any part of the plant may cause a burning sensation on the skin.

Poisoning, with similar symptoms, has occurred in cattle and horses, but more commonly in pigs after eating the roots. Inflammation of the eyes, staggering and paralysis have been reported in pigs.

Removal of plant material from the stomach is necessary only in the case of small children or if a large number of berries have been eaten. In such cases medical advice should be sought.

POLYGONACEAE

In addition to the familiar rhubarb, the leaves of which can cause poisoning (see below), this family contains some other cultivated and wild plants which are potentially toxic (see list, page 104).

Rhubarb *Rheum rhaponticum* (photo 58)

This perennial plant is commonly grown in gardens because the long, pinkish-red stalks of the leaves are edible when cooked; without adequate sweetening, stewed rhubarb is very sour. Leaves grow from 'crowns' just below the surface of the ground and, when fully expanded, each leaf blade can be 30–60 cm (1–2 ft) across. They are somewhat triangular in outline, but have an undulating, slightly wavy edge. When young, the leaves are bright green, shiny and crinkled. Small, creamy-red flowers sometimes develop in densely crowded masses on erect, hollow, jointed, reddish stems.

• **POISONOUS SUBSTANCES** There are oxalates in all parts of the plant, particularly the leaves. Oxalates combine with calcium in the blood. This results in a reduction in the calcium content of the blood and the formation of calcium oxalate crystals in various parts of the body. Anthraquinone glycosides are also present and may be responsible for some toxicity.

• **POISONING** There is no danger in eating the red leaf stalks of rhubarb when cooked, but many cases of poisoning have arisen from eating the leaves. In the First World War, when this practice was recommended in Britain, there were even some deaths. Within an hour of eating rhubarb leaves there can be nausea, stomach pains, vomiting, weakness and drowsiness; muscular twitching and convulsions may follow. Blood clotting is impaired and there may be haemorrhages. It is unwise to eat any part of rhubarb raw; apart from digestive-system disturbances, liver and kidney damage may result.

Under normal conditions, animals do not have access to rhubarb, but it is dangerous to give them discarded leaves; poisoning, sometimes fatal, has been reported in cattle, pigs, goats and poultry. The symptoms are similar to those of human poisoning; affected animals may also foam at the mouth and have severe diarrhoea.

Professional treatment is required in all but mild cases, as it may be necessary to give injections of calcium preparations.

RANUNCULACEAE

Many members of this large family have a bitter taste and so are generally avoided, although some, such as anemones, buttercups and clematis (see below) have caused poisoning if eaten in quantity. Also in this family are the monkshoods (*Aconitum* species), which are particularly dangerous (see below). For other potentially poisonous garden plants see list, page 105.

Monkshood *Aconitum napellus* (photo 59)

There are several slightly different forms of monkshood, the one that still grows wild in a very few localities in the south-west of Britain often being called *Aconitum anglicum*. The ones most likely to be seen are garden varieties. Monkshood is similar to the related plant, delphinium. It is a perennial, with thick, blackish roots, leaves up to 15 cm (6 in) long and a tall flowering stem up to 1 m (3 ft) high. The leaves have three to five deeply divided segments, with irregular edges and pointed teeth. The flowers are a deep blue, although some varieties have paler blue, or purple flowers; each is hooded or helmet shaped, with the upper segments curving down over the lower ones.

• POISONOUS SUBSTANCES All parts of the plant contain aconitine and other similar alkaloids. The alkaloid content varies considerably with soil type and season; in winter the roots are particularly poisonous. At least some of the toxins remain after drying or storage.

• POISONING Monkshood is one of the most poisonous plants known, as even small amounts can cause severe or fatal poisoning. Incidents of poisoning are, however, very rare: it is extremely unpalatable, publicity is given to its toxicity and, in Britain, it is not a common plant. Symptoms of poisoning develop in less than an hour. Initially there is a burning sensation in the mouth and throat; both coldness and sweating are experienced. Later symptoms include a general numbness, vomiting and diarrhoea with severe abdominal pain. The final stages are characterized by slow pulse, convulsions and sometimes coma. Death may occur within two hours.

Cattle and horses have shown symptoms similar to those of human poisoning, but, in general, poisoning of animals by monkshood is rare. It should, however, be considered a dangerous plant for all animals and they should not be allowed to eat it in any form.

Professional advice should be sought urgently if monkshood poisoning is suspected.

• NOTE Particular care should be taken when disposing of garden rubbish containing these plants.

Wood Anemone *Anemone nemorosa* (photo 60)

This perennial, spring-flowering plant occurs throughout most of Britain as ground cover in deciduous woods on all but the most acid or water-logged soils. The flower stalk grows from a brown, underground stem and bears a single ring of three, stalked leaves, which are deeply divided into delicate, pointed segments with serrated edges. The flowers are borne singly and are held on a slender stalk among or above the leaves. There are usually six or seven, rounded, petal-like segments, curving slightly inwards around a central cluster of numerous stamens. The flowers are usually white or pinkish, but may be tinged with blue. After flowering, more leaves, similar to those on the flower stalk, develop from ground level.

• POISONOUS SUBSTANCE The glycoside ranunculin, from which the volatile oil, protoanemonin, is formed, is present at its highest concentration in the leaves and sap of the plant during flowering; the unearthed roots can also be dangerous. It is unstable and the dried plant is not poisonous.

• POISONING It is unlikely that people would eat wood anemones, but damage to the mouth and all other parts of the digestive system could occur. If the sap comes in contact with the skin it can cause reddening and blister formation.

Because of its acrid taste, it is generally not eaten by animals, although this may happen in early spring when other green feed is scarce. Protoanemonin is an irritant that causes inflammation of the mouth, salivation and abdominal pain. This may be followed by ulceration in the mouth and damage to the digestive and urinary systems.

Poisoning is generally not severe enough to require more treatment than administration of soothing drinks.

• NOTE Other *Anemone* species, such as *Anemone coronaria*, often sold by florists, and the pasque flower *(Pulsatilla vulgaris)*, grown in gardens and occasionally found wild, are also potentially poisonous, as they, too, contain protoanemonin. Actual cases of poisoning by these plants are, however, rare.

Traveller's Joy *Clematis vitalba* (photo 62)
Old Man's Beard

This is a common climbing plant found mainly on chalky soils. It is perennial and has stems that grow up to 30 m (100 ft) long; often these almost cover the trees and shrubs over which they climb. The stems are woody at the base, with a fibrous outer layer that sometimes hangs off in shreds. Higher up, the stems are green and bear leaves with winding stalks. Each leaf has usually five widely separated leaflets that are oval or pointed and up to 10 cm (4 in) long. Clusters of small, stalked, yellowish-white flowers develop in summer; in autumn the characteristic 'old man's beard' is apparent, as the fruits have long, curved, whitish, feathery plumes.

• POISONOUS SUBSTANCE The whole plant contains the glycoside ranunculin, from which protoanemonin, an irritant substance, is formed; this substance is no longer present in the plant when dried.

• POISONING The toxicity of this plant is generally considered to be only slight, and there have been no reports found of human poisoning, although the sap can cause blistering of the skin.

Animals generally do not eat *Clematis*, presumably because of its bitter taste and burning effect in the mouth. There is, however, a report of fatal poisoning in a cow that developed noisy breathing, sore eyes, and ulceration of the muzzle after eating the plant. It showed signs of abdominal pain, became weak, and died within a few hours.

• NOTE Garden varieties of *Clematis* are also said to contain the same toxins, but there is no detailed information available. It is, therefore, advisable to treat them all with caution, to avoid skin contact, and not to allow animals access to them.

Buttercup *Ranunculus* species (photo 63)

Several species of buttercup and of the closely related plants, such as crowfoot, spearwort and marsh marigold, are common throughout Britain, many occurring in damp places. The leaves of most have three main lobes or leaflets, each deeply indented and irregularly toothed, giving a somewhat delicate appearance. The flowers of most are yellow, about 2 cm (¾ in) across, with usually five rounded petals forming a shallow cup around the mass of yellow, pollen-bearing stamens in the centre. The crowfoots, which have white flowers, grow mainly in water; most have some floating leaves with rounded lobes and some submerged leaves that are finely divided into slender threads.

• POISONOUS SUBSTANCE All parts of these plants contain the glycoside ranunculin, from which the irritant substance protoanemonin is formed. The highest concentration is present at the time of flowering. Protoanemonin is unstable, so that hay containing buttercups is safe to feed to animals.

• POISONING The plants in this group vary in their toxicity. Their bitter, burning taste is a deterrent to their being eaten. None is likely to cause human poisoning except in unusual circumstances; the bulbous base of *Ranunculus bulbosus* has caused poisoning in children when mistaken for the underground parts of edible plants. When these plants have been eaten, digestive-system disturbances have occurred.

Animals also tend not to eat the plants in pasture, but where they are abundant, this is unavoidable. The celery-leaved buttercup (*Ranunculus sceleratus*) is responsible for most cases of poisoning, but it may be that, because of its vigorous growth, it is eaten in larger amounts. There is a danger of poisoning when plants are cut and fed fresh to housed animals, but not when cut and dried before feeding.

All domestic animals appear to be susceptible to protoanemonin poisoning and a variety of symptoms have been attributed to eating plants containing it. In general, however, there is excessive flow of saliva, soreness (sometimes with ulceration) of the mouth, and abdominal pain. In severe cases, this is followed by diarrhoea, blood-stained urine, staggering and sometimes impaired hearing and sight. In the few animals that die, convulsions often precede death.

Treatment is necessary only in severe cases.

● NOTE After the use of weed-killers, buttercups appear to be more palatable and are more readily consumed by animals, so that there is a greater risk of poisoning. It is generally recommended that treated pastures should not be grazed for at least 14 days after the application of herbicides.

RHAMNACEAE

Most members of this family are trees or shrubs, two of which are native to Britain and poisonous: alder buckthorn *(Frangula alnus)* and buckthorn *(Rhamnus cathartica)*.

Alder Buckthorn *Frangula alnus*

This shrub, still often called by its former name, *Rhamnus frangula*, is generally not common but grows throughout Britain on damp peaty soils. The shrub is thornless and grows 4–5 m (13–16 ft) tall. The branches point upwards, close to the trunk and the bark is generally smooth. The oval, pointed leaves are shiny and green, becoming yellow or red in autumn. The flowers are greenish white and the fruits change from red to purplish black when ripe. For details of poisoning see under buckthorn below.

Buckthorn *Rhamnus cathartica* (photo 64)

Buckthorn grows in scrub, hedges and beneath larger trees in woods, mainly on chalky soils. It forms a thorny shrub or small tree, usually 4–6 m (13–20 ft) tall. The bark on old trees is often split and scaly, with an orange tinge. The branches spread almost at right angles to the trunk. The young twigs may be softly hairy or smooth and bear stalked, oval leaves that are dull green and turn yellowish brown in autumn. The inconspicuous greenish-white flowers develop into green fruits, usually just over 0.5 cm (less than 0.5 in) across, which ripen from red to black. There are several cultivated varieties, some of which are variegated and thornless.

● POISONOUS SUBSTANCES The buckthorns contain anthraquinone glycosides from which toxic anthraquinones are liberated.

● **POISONING** Children sometimes eat the berries or chew the twigs. If a few berries are eaten there is only mild stomach ache, perhaps with vomiting and diarrhoea, but if large quantities are eaten, there may be severe digestive-system symptoms with haemorrhage followed by convulsions, difficult breathing and even death.

Buckthorn poisoning is rare in animals, but diarrhoea and violent vomiting were reported in a cow that ate leaves, twigs and fruit (with seeds) of alder buckthorn; it died within a few hours. Diarrhoea and abdominal pain were reported recently in horses after alder buckthorn branches with berries were thrown onto their pasture; symptoms subsided in 2–8 days.

Professional advice should be sought as poisoning can be severe.

● **NOTE** The purgative properties of plants in this family have long been known; the well known laxative cascara is prepared from the bark of the North American shrub *Rhamnus purshiana*.

ROSACEAE

Some of the many members of this family present in Britain can cause cyanide poisoning, the kernels within the fruits having a potentially high cyanide content. The cherry laurel *(Prunus laurocerasus)*, however, is the most frequent cause of poisoning. For others see list, page 106.

Cherry Laurel *Prunus laurocerasus* (photo 65)
Laurel

The common name, laurel, could lead to confusion with other plants, such as spurge laurel or wood laurel, which are also poisonous. These are *Daphne* species and belong to another plant family, Thymelaeaceae.

This evergreen shrub is not native in Britain, but is often planted in shrubberies or used for hedging. The seeds may be dispersed, and self-sown bushes (apparently naturalized) are not infrequent. Laurel is a vigorously growing shrub or small tree up to 6 m (20 ft) high, with well developed branches. These have dark, greyish-brown bark, and bear oval, short-stalked leaves that are bright green and glossy when young, but tough, leathery and darker green later. Each leaf is about 10 cm (4 in) long and smooth edged. Erect spikes of creamy-white flowers can be seen in early summer, and develop into bunches of oval or spherical, purplish-black, juicy berries in autumn.

● **POISONOUS SUBSTANCES** Cyanogenic glycosides (prunasin and amygdalin) are present in varying amounts in the leaves and the seeds of the fruits.

● **POISONING** Human poisoning is rare, but children may find the berries attractive and eat them. The flesh is relatively harmless, but serious or even fatal poisoning can result if the seeds are chewed. Mistaken use of laurel leaves instead of bay leaves as food flavouring can also cause poisoning. Symptoms develop within a few hours and include vomiting, flushing of the cheeks, rapid breathing, headache, fainting, and convulsions; unless treatment is started quickly, the patient may die.

Although all animals are susceptible to poisoning by laurel *(Prunus* species), they rarely eat them. When they do, however, sudden death may result; in less severe cases the symptoms include rapid breathing, dilatation of pupils, trembling, staggering and sometimes falling and convulsions. The lining of the mouth is bright red initially, becoming bluish later. The flesh of poisoned animals often smells of almonds; it should not be fed to other animals.

Poisoning can be rapidly fatal and professional advice should be sought urgently. Specific treatment for cyanide poisoning is available and, if given early enough, can be successful even in severe cases.

● **NOTE** Other members of this family can also cause cyanide poisoning. Portugal laurel *(Prunus lusitanica)* caused severe diarrhoea, shivering and trembling in a young goat that broke into a garden. Two goats that ate the leaves and fruit of a crab-apple tree *(Malus sylvestris)* developed symptoms typical of cyanide poisoning; one died and one recovered after treatment. The kernels and pips in the fruits of some members of the Rosaceae family contain high levels of cyanogenic glycosides. Human poisoning has resulted from eating bitter almonds, apricot kernels or a large quantity of apple pips, and pigs have been poisoned when plum stones, removed during jam making, or discarded plums from a heavy crop were added to their feed.

SCROPHULARIACEAE

This large family includes quite a number of wild plants found in Britain, many of which have cultivated forms grown in gardens. One of these that has long been recognized to be poisonous is the foxglove *(Digitalis purpurea)*. For a few others suspected of being poisonous see list, page 107.

Foxglove *Digitalis purpurea* (photo 66)

This widely distributed plant is common in woodland clearings, heaths, hillsides and hedgerows. The wild plant and cultivated varieties are also grown in gardens. At ground level there are large, coarse-textured, hairy leaves,

15–30 cm (6–12 in) long. The flower spike, which grows in the second year, can be up to 1.5 m (5 ft) tall. The flowers hang down close together on the stem and open in succession from the base up. They are pinkish purple and tubular in shape, with a protruding lower lip on which there are numerous small dark spots, often within white circles. Bumble bees alight on the lip and crawl in to pollinate the flowers.

● POISONOUS SUBSTANCES Glycosides, such as digitoxin and digitalin that affect the action of the heart, are present in the whole plant; drying, storage or boiling do not reduce its toxicity.

● POISONING The bitter taste of this plant is a deterrent to its being eaten, but human poisoning has occurred after eating leaves or flowers, or drinking tea prepared from the leaves. The symptoms include nausea, vomiting (sometimes persisting for more than 24 hours), abdominal pain, diarrhoea, headache, and slow irregular pulse. In more severe cases, disturbances of vision, trembling, convulsions, delirium, and hallucinations can also develop. Large amounts of toxin are rarely absorbed because vomiting usually occurs.

Poisoning has been reported, although infrequently, in most domestic animals. The symptoms are similar to those in human poisoning, with diarrhoea, abdominal pain, irregular pulse, trembling and convulsions. Animals sometimes develop a craving for the plant.

For treatment, vomiting should be induced and professional advice sought.

● NOTE In 1785 a book by an English doctor, William Withering, was published on medicinal uses of foxglove preparations; today several drugs derived from the plant are still in use, particularly for the treatment of heart conditions. Yellow halos around objects have been seen after excessive use of medicinal preparations, and it has been suggested that the prominence of yellow in Van Gogh's late paintings could be attributed to his having been given digitalis treatment.

SOLANACEAE

Although this large family does contain some important edible plants, such as the potato and tomato, many of its members are poisonous, including all those native to Britain (the nightshades and henbane) and two introduced species (thorn apple and the Duke of Argyll's tea plant), both occasionally found growing wild. Some poisonous garden and house plants (see list, page 108) also belong to this family.

Deadly Nightshade *Atropa belladonna* (photo 67)

This plant is rather rare in the country as a whole, but is fairly common within some limited areas, scattered among trees and at the edge of woods on chalky soils in south-east England. It is a large plant, up to 1.5 m (5 ft) high, with erect branching stems giving it a bushy appearance. The stems grow each year from the perennial rootstock, and bear oval, pointed leaves on alternate sides of the stem, singly or in pairs of unequal size. The flower buds are upright, but the flowers tend to droop on their stalks. They grow singly or in pairs in the axils of the leaves or in the forks of the branches. When fully developed the flowers are elongated, up to 3 cm (1¼ in) long and bell shaped, the lower edge having five pointed lobes. The outer side of the flower is usually greenish, but the inside is a dull purple or brownish red. The fruits are shiny, black berries, with the five green, pointed lobes that enclosed the bud partly surrounding the base.

• POISONOUS SUBSTANCES All parts of the plant, but particularly the berries, contain a variable mixture of tropane alkaloids: hyoscyamine, hyoscine (scopolamine), atropine. The alkaloid composition changes during drying, but the plant is still poisonous.

• POISONING This has sometimes resulted from misidentification of the plant when the leafy part has been cooked and eaten as a vegetable or the berries stewed for a dessert. Most cases, however, involve children who pick and eat the berries direct from the plant; five berries or less have caused severe or fatal poisoning in young children. Eating deadly nightshade berries is always harmful. The symptoms develop within a few hours and include dry mouth, flushing of the face, dilatation of the pupils and a rapid pulse. There may be difficulty in breathing, digestive disturbances (usually constipation), convulsions, hallucinations and coma; without treatment, death may follow within 6–24 hours. The sap of the plant can cause soreness and blistering of the skin.

Most animals are susceptible to deadly nightshade poisoning, although some, such as rabbits, are more resistant; other animals or people eating their flesh, can, however, be poisoned. Poisoning in animals does not occur very frequently, but fatal cases have been reported: in calves after eating the plants growing in a neglected garden, in pigs that ate the plants during a drought, and in a goat which developed typical symptoms, with continuous crying before dying. The symptoms are similar in all animals and resemble those of human poisoning.

If deadly nightshade poisoning is suspected, professional advice should be sought urgently; it may be necessary to remove stomach contents.

• NOTE As its name suggests, this is the most poisonous of the nightshades. Woody nightshade *(Solanum dulcamara)*, with small purple flowers and berries that are red when ripe (see page 79) is often incorrectly called deadly nightshade.

Thorn Apple *Datura stramonium* (photo 68)
Jimsonweed

This plant is not common in Britain, but has become established in some areas, mainly in waste places, roadsides, and railway embankments; some species of *Datura* are cultivated in gardens or glasshouses. Thorn apple is a large annual, with forked branches, growing up to 1 m (3 ft) high. The leaves are up to 20 cm (8 in) long, irregularly pointed at the edges and sometimes yellowish near the base, especially when young. The flowers appear singly as erect, white or purplish trumpets up to 10 cm (4 in) long. The fruits are green, spiny, oval or spherical capsules, 2–5 cm (1–2 in) long, that split from the apex into four segments, revealing the numerous, wrinkled black seeds. The plant has a distinctive, unpleasant odour, especially when bruised or crushed.

• POISONOUS SUBSTANCES The whole plant, especially the flowers and seeds, contains toxic tropane alkaloids, whose concentration can vary considerably with stage of growth and environmental conditions. The toxicity of the plant is due mainly to the alkaloids hyoscyamine and hyoscine (scopolamine) that are also present in deadly nightshade and are closely related to atropine; their activity is not eliminated by drying or boiling. Nitrates may also be present.

• POISONING Thorn apple preparations have been used medicinally for many centuries, and the influence of the plant on human behaviour is well documented. It is through using the plant to produce hallucinogenic effects that most cases of poisoning occur. In addition, children may be attracted by the trumpet-shaped flowers or the spiny fruits and eat them or the seeds within them. Within an hour or two the mouth becomes dry, the skin flushed and the pupils dilated. There may be feelings of nausea and drowsiness, with a rise in temperature and, depending on the amount taken, agitation, rapid or irregular heart beat and hallucinations, leading to highly abnormal behaviour. This state can be followed by delirium, convulsions, coma and sometimes death. Visual disturbances may persist for up to two weeks.

Animals are unlikely to eat the growing plant, but may consume the dried plant in hay, or the seeds in grain feed. Poisoning has been recorded in all types of farm animal, with symptoms similar to those seen in human poisoning. Piglets with joint abnormalities have been born to sows that have eaten the plant during pregnancy.

Professional treatment is essential and hospital care may be needed.

• NOTE As thorn apple is not a common plant in this country, poisoning is infrequent but can be severe. Roman soldiers were poisoned by the plant around 38 BC; the name Jimsonweed originated when poisoning occurred among soldiers at Jamestown, USA, in 1676, and soldiers again were involved in a mass outbreak of poisoning in North Africa in 1943. These incidents emphasize the potential danger of eating wild plants.

Henbane *Hyoscyamus niger* (photo 69)

This distinctive plant, once found in some areas along the sandy coast of Britain, is now seen only occasionally in such places. It may also be found on waste land near the coast or near old buildings (where it was grown in former times for medicinal purposes). Henbane is a sturdy plant, up to 75 cm (2½ ft) high, with a thick stem and lobed or toothed leaves. Those near the base are stalked, but higher up they have no stalks and are crowded together near the stem. The whole plant is hairy, somewhat sticky and has a strong, unpleasant smell. The flowers form in clusters near the top of the stems, bending downwards when in bud, but pointing upwards when open. They are funnel-shaped, up to 3 cm (1¼ in) across, and whitish or yellowish, with prominent purple veins; the inner part of the flower is often uniformly purple. The green covering of the bud grows up around the fruit, its five points hardening into spines.

- POISONOUS SUBSTANCES The whole plant, including the seeds, contains a mixture of alkaloids, the main ones being hyoscyamine and hyoscine (scopolamine), also present in deadly nightshade; their toxicity remains after drying.

- POISONING As henbane is uncommon in this country and has an unpleasant taste, it rarely causes poisoning. It is, however, a dangerously poisonous plant with an action similar to that of deadly nightshade. The thick roots have been mistaken for those of edible wild plants, the leaves have been used in salads, and the flowers eaten for their hallucinogenic properties. A 20-year-old man who chewed four flowers to produce an intended pleasant sensation was found lying on a footpath; be became excitable and restless, with a rapid pulse and hot dry skin, and had difficulty in seeing and swallowing. He experienced hallucinations and behaved in a bizarre manner; recovery was complete in 48 hours. Mild symptoms, including dry mouth, blurred vision, mental confusion, and dilated pupils, may be followed by more serious ones, such as loud, rapid heart beat, staggering, extreme agitation, unconsciousness, hallucinations and even death.

Animals seldom graze the plant in its natural state, but cattle have been poisoned by henbane contained in hay or in cut green feed, and pigs have also been poisoned. In addition to the symptoms in human poisoning, the animals developed convulsions before death.

The serious nature of henbane poisoning necessitates urgent professional care.

Christmas Cherry
Solanum capsicastrum and *Solanum pseudocapsicum* (photo 71)
Winter Cherry; Jerusalem Cherry; Capsicum

These plants are very similar, share the same common names and are often confused with each other. In Britain they are grown as house plants and are especially popular at Christmas time, when the red berries are present. They are small, woody shrubs with branches bearing dark-green, narrow, pointed leaves. *Solanum capsicastrum* has smooth, wavy leaves and slightly hairy stems; *Solanum pseudocapsicum* has soft, velvety leaves, hairless stems and is a slightly more vigorous plant. A profusion of small white flowers with pointed petals and yellowish centres (stamens) grows in summer. The fruits, which form from these, ripen from green, through yellow to orange or bright shiny red, depending on the variety. They are not related to true (edible) cherries, as their common names could imply.

- **POISONOUS SUBSTANCE** An alkaloid solanocapsine is present in all parts of the plants, including the fruits.

- **POISONING** Children find the fruits attractive and may be tempted to eat them. The effects are not serious, but eating even a few can result in nausea, abdominal pain and drowsiness.

There are no reports of poisoning in animals, but it would be wise to keep these plants out of the reach of pets that are likely to eat them.

- **NOTE** The related chilli pepper *(Capsicum annuum)* is sometimes grown in gardens, glasshouses or indoors. As the attractive, elongated, cone-shaped fruits ripen they change from green to yellowish-orange and finally to bright red. They make popular house plants, particularly at Christmas, or the pods may be used as a hot flavouring for food. If eaten mistakenly or by children attracted by their bright colours, they produce an intense burning sensation in the mouth and throat, but are otherwise harmless.

Woody Nightshade *Solanum dulcamara*
(photos 70 and 72)
Bittersweet

This perennial plant has long, trailing stems that grow from the woody base each spring. They may be up to 3 m (10 ft) long and scramble over and through trees and hedges or, particularly in coastal areas, spread along the ground. The dark-green leaves are pointed, and often have small, stalked leaflets or lobes near the base. The loosely clustered flowers are on branched stalks; they are about 1 cm (⅓ in) across, and have purple petals surrounding a prominent yellow centre, composed of a 'cone' of stamens. The oval fruits ripen from green to shiny red in autumn.

● **POISONOUS SUBSTANCE** The whole plant contains the alkaloid solanine, whose concentration is highest in the unripe green berries and lowest in the ripe red berries.

● **POISONING** Human poisoning is usually associated with eating the berries; when ripe and red they are particularly attractive to children. As these are the least poisonous part of the plant, there are often no symptoms at all or only mild stomach pains. If eaten in large numbers or when green, however, more serious symptoms can occur, as in the case of a nine-year-old girl who died, in England, in 1948. In addition to stomach pains her symptoms included vomiting, thirst, distressed breathing and exhaustion.

This plant is not a common cause of poisoning in animals, but there are old reports involving cattle and sheep. In one outbreak in cattle, the symptoms included muscular tremors, falling, a rapid pulse and subnormal temperature. Diarrhoea, staggering and falling, increased temperature and rate of breathing, feeble pulse and some deaths have been reported in sheep.

In all but the mildest cases, professional advice should be sought.

● **NOTE** Because of the similarities in names, this plant can be confused with deadly nightshade and black nightshade.

Black Nightshade *Solanum nigrum* (photo 73)
Garden Nightshade

Black nightshade is common on wasteland and in coastal areas. It also grows as a weed in agricultural land and gardens throughout the country, except in Scotland where it is rare. Because it can grow in such profusion it is becoming a serious problem in some areas, particularly as the poisonous berries are likely to be harvested with food crops, such as peas. In agricultural land, weed-killers often cannot be used, as the black nightshade and the crop grow together; there is also evidence that the plant is developing resistance to some weed-killers. This plant varies in size and form, according to where it is growing; it may be small, barely 15 cm (6 in) high and lie close to the ground, or develop into a thriving, bushy plant up to 60 cm (2 ft) high. The branching stems bear oval or diamond-shaped leaves, sometimes with wavy or toothed edges, and, in summer, clusters of small flowers. The pointed, white petals tend to turn back in older flowers. The ripe fruits are shiny, black, spherical berries that contain numerous seeds.

● **POISONOUS SUBSTANCES** The whole plant contains various glycoalkaloids, including solanine, with highest concentrations in the unripe green berries and lowest in the roots. The great variation in the alkaloid content of black nightshade has led to conflicting reports about its toxicity. In silage the plant is less poisonous. Nitrates in the plant may contribute to its toxic effects.

• POISONING This usually results from the berries being eaten. If these are ripe, there may be no or only very mild symptoms, but the unripe berries can cause vomiting, diarrhoea, headache, dizziness and increase in body temperature; these usually start within about eight hours. In severe cases, there can be coma and even death.

Black nightshade is sometimes harvested with crops and inadvertently fed to farm animals; they will also occasionally eat the growing plant. Signs of poisoning include difficulty in breathing, various digestive-system disturbances (vomiting, abdominal pain, constipation, diarrhoea), dilated pupils, and loss of coordination; severely affected animals may die.

Professional treatment is required.

Potato *Solanum tuberosum* (photo 74)

This plant originated in South America, but is now cultivated throughout most of the world for its edible underground tubers, potatoes. In spring these develop green shoots, which grow rapidly to form tough, often straggling stems up to 1 m (3 ft) long. The leaves grow along these stems with a single leaflet, often the largest, at the tip and two lateral rows of broad oval leaflets, interspersed with varying numbers of smaller leaflets. The five-pointed flowers appear in late spring and are white, pale purple or tinged with red, depending on the variety. After flowering, many varieties of potato, particularly some of the newer ones, produce small, round fruits, rather like green tomatoes. The tubers are produced on whitish underground stems.

• POISONOUS SUBSTANCES All parts of the plant growing above the ground, and particularly the fruits, contain alkaloids, the most important of which is solanine. It is only after prolonged exposure to light or unsuitable storage that the potato tubers contain sufficient solanine to be poisonous. Nitrates present in potato foliage may contribute to poisoning in animals.

• POISONING The tomato-like fruits can be attractive to children. The day after eating potato fruit (amount not known) a sixteen-month-old boy developed abdominal pain and vomiting; eating large quantities can be dangerous. Potatoes that have sprouted or been left in the light and become green usually contain high concentrations of solanine and are therefore not safe to eat, even after peeling and cooking. Symptoms vary from mild digestive disturbances, often not attributed to potatoes, to much more severe illness, as in the incident in south-east London involving 78 schoolboys in 1969. At the beginning of the autumn term they were given potatoes from a bag that had been left over at the end of the summer term. About eight to ten hours after the meal, they developed abdominal pain, vomiting and diarrhoea.

81

In some boys this was followed by drowsiness, delirium, hallucinations, aching limbs, restlessness, and unconsciousness; 17 boys were admitted to hospital, three being extremely ill. All eventually recovered.

Poisoning in farm animals can be caused by feeding them with leaves and stems of the plant, or waste, rotting or sprouted potatoes not considered fit for human food. Symptoms similar to those described for human poisoning have been reported in cattle and pigs; sudden death has also occurred in some outbreaks in pigs. Other animals, including sheep and horses, have also been affected, and a dog that became lethargic and then unconscious was found to have ten small green potatoes in its stomach.

If more than mild vomiting and diarrhoea occur, professional advice should be sought.

● **NOTE** To avoid production of solanine, potatoes should always be stored in the dark; sprouting potatoes should not be eaten.

TAXACEAE

This family of evergreen trees and shrubs contains only one British species, which is highly poisonous, the yew *(Taxus baccata)*. Other *Taxus* species, planted in parks and gardens, have also been reported to be similarly poisonous.

Yew *Taxus baccata* (photo 75)

In its natural state, the English yew is a spreading evergreen tree growing up to 20 m (65 ft) tall and often living for many hundreds of years. It can be found throughout the country, but mainly on chalk or limestone. An upright form, the Irish yew, and ornamentals such as the Japanese yew *(Taxus cuspidata)* also grow in Britain. Yews are planted in parks and gardens and are a feature of some churchyards; they are often used for hedging. The bark is reddish brown, scaly, fibrous and may be deeply fissured. The small, elongated, narrow leaves, up to 3 cm (1¼ in) long and 4 mm (⅛ in) wide, are crowded together on the twigs. The short stalks of the English yew twist so that the leaves lie more or less in one plane; they are dark green and glossy above and paler beneath. The male and female flowers are usually on separate trees. The conspicuous pinkish-red fruits develop in autumn as fleshy cups surrounding the seeds on the female trees.

● **POISONOUS SUBSTANCES** A mixture of alkaloids (taxines) are present in all parts of the plant except the fleshy red part of the fruit. The toxicity is not decreased in fallen branches or hedge trimmings.

• **POISONING** Fatal human poisoning has occurred after eating the leaves or fruits, the latter being particularly attractive to children. The fruits cause poisoning only if the seeds within them are chewed. The toxic alkaloids are then released and produce effects that range from mild nausea and abdominal pain to coma and death. These alkaloids are absorbed rapidly from the digestive tract and interfere with the action of the heart. In many cases there is sudden collapse, followed by death; in others, this may be preceded by lethargy, trembling, staggering, coldness, dilatation of the pupils, a rapid then weak pulse, and convulsions.

Poisoning has been reported in many different farm and zoo animals. Farmers are generally well aware of the highly poisonous nature of yew, and most cases in farm animals occur in special circumstances, such as when fences are broken, giving access to the trees; in winter, when food is scarce or branches are weighed down by snow to within the reach of the animals; and when branches fall or hedge cuttings are thrown onto pasture. Death may be so sudden that animals, particularly cattle, are just found dead, with diagnosis being made only on the presence of yew in the stomach or still in the mouth. Poisoning is not always as sudden as this, however, and symptoms similar to those of human poisoning may be seen for three or four days before death or, in some cases, recovery. Birds may eat the fruits without any apparent ill effects; this is because the red fleshy part of the fruit is harmless and the hard poisonous seed passes undamaged through the digestive system. Pheasants have been poisoned by eating the leaves.

Because of the possibility of fatal poisoning, professional advice should be sought at once.

THYMELAEACEAE

Two shrubs of this family are native to Britain: the spurge laurel *(Daphne laureola)* and mezereon *(Daphne mezereum)*. Both produce a similar type of poisoning (see below). They, as well as other *Daphne* species, are also cultivated in gardens. Little is known, however, about the toxicity of the cultivated species and varieties.

Spurge Laurel *Daphne laureola* (photo 77)
Wood Laurel

Although not abundant, spurge laurel is found growing wild in Britain, usually in woods on chalky soils. It is not unusual to find it growing singly rather than in groups. Spurge laurel is an evergreen shrub, up to 1 m (3 ft) tall. The dark-green, glossy leaves are up to 12.5 cm (5 in) long and widen to 1 cm (⅓ in) near the tip, before terminating in a blunt point. The greenish flowers develop in short spikes from where the leaf stalks join the main stems. The fruit, an oval berry, is green at first but blue black when ripe. For details of poisoning see under mezereon below.

Mezereon *Daphne mezereum* (photo 76)

It is now very rare to find this small shrub growing wild in Britain, but there are several garden varieties. The woody, upright twigs bear fragrant flowers in spring, before the leaves develop. The leaves are small, usually less than 10 cm (4 in) long, and are narrow, with a pointed tip. At first they are pale green, but darken when fully grown. The flowers are produced in small clusters and are usually white or shades of pink; in autumn they develop into bright-red, oval berries.

• POISONOUS SUBSTANCES Several substances in these plants have been identified and named, some of them as possible toxins, but two diterpene esters, mezerein and daphnetoxin, are now thought to be the major ones. All parts of the plants are poisonous, especially the seeds in the berries; their toxicity is not destroyed by drying and storage.

• POISONING This is uncommon, but when it does occur it is usually caused by eating mezereon or spurge laurel berries, which resemble red or black currants, respectively, and are attractive to children. These have an acrid taste, however, so that generally only a few are eaten, although only one may be enough to produce some mild, transient symptoms, including a burning sensation in the mouth, nausea, vomiting, stomach pains and diarrhoea. A few berries are sufficient to cause severe forms of these symptoms, with weakness, disorientation, and convulsions, followed by death.

Animals generally avoid the plants, although young pigs have been killed by placing as few as three berries per pig in their feeding trough. The symptoms are similar to those described in human poisoning.

These plants are dangerously poisonous and professional attention should be sought immediately if poisoning is suspected.

• NOTE The common names of *Daphne laureola* sometimes lead to confusion with other unrelated laurels, *Prunus* species, in the Rosaceae family. It is important to identify them accurately, as the two types of plant contain different poisonous substances.

UMBELLIFERAE

This family contains several well-known food plants such as carrots, celery and parsley, but also includes some of the most poisonous plants found in Britain;

cowbane *(Cicuta virosa)*, hemlock *(Conium maculatum)*, and hemlock water dropwort *(Oenanthe crocata)*. A few other wild plants in the family that are less toxic are listed on page 109. Contact with some of the wild and cultivated Umbelliferae can cause damage to skin exposed to bright sunlight; giant hogweed *(Heracleum mantegazzianum)* is the best known of these, and others are listed on page 109.

Cowbane *Cicuta virosa* (photo 78)

This plant is found in only a few isolated parts of Britain, but may be quite common within these areas. It grows in shallow water, ditches and beside ponds, mainly in East Anglia, but also in the west Midlands and southern Scotland. Cowbane is a strong, erect plant with smooth, hollow, finely ridged stems up to 1.5 m (5 ft) tall. The leaves are divided into leaflets, each of which is further divided into elongated, narrow lobes, pointed at the tip and serrated at the edges. The flower heads (umbels) are 7.5–15 cm (3–6 in) across and are composed of 10–30 rounded groups of small white flowers, each group growing on a slender stalk (ray) from the top of the stem. The rootstock of cowbane is characteristic, being elongated, thick, white and fleshy, with a partially hollow centre, crossed at intervals by thin partitions.

• POISONOUS SUBSTANCE An unsaturated higher alcohol, cicutoxin, is present in all parts of the plant, particularly in the yellow juice of the underground parts; it is still active in the dried plant.

• POISONING As cowbane is an uncommon plant in Britain, instances of poisoning are rare, although it is extremely poisonous. The plant can easily be confused with edible plants of the same family, such as wild carrot or wild parsnip; even a few bites of the misidentified plant can cause serious poisoning or death. Symptoms may be noticed within half an hour of eating cowbane. Initially there is burning of the mouth, profuse production of saliva, nausea and vomiting, but no diarrhoea; flushing, dizziness, dilatation of pupils, and, later a bluish tinge of the skin are often reported. Muscular contractions and convulsions, accompanied by difficulty in breathing, are followed by unconsciousness and death, often within a few hours of eating the plant.

Animals are most at risk when soil disturbance has exposed the underground parts of the plant. The symptoms are similar to those of human poisoning.

Professional help should be sought as quickly as possible to control the convulsions and assist breathing.

• NOTE Cowbane is a dangerously poisonous plant as even small quantities can cause fatal poisoning.

Hemlock *Conium maculatum* (photo 79)

Hemlock grows throughout Britain, but is infrequent in the north. It is generally associated with damp places, but is also commonly found on roadsides and at the edges of fields. The plant grows up to 2 m (6½ ft) tall and has a delicate appearance, due to the very finely divided, fern-like leaves. Characteristic features of hemlock are the irregular purple blotches on the smooth, hollow stem, and the generally mousy smell that is especially obvious when the leaves or flowers are crushed. Small, white flowers are produced, crowded together into rounded clusters, 10–20 of which arise together on slender stalks forming a group, the 'umbel', at the top of the stem or its branches.

• POISONOUS SUBSTANCES Coniine, gamma-coniceine and other related alkaloids are present in varying concentrations in the whole plant. Much of the toxicity is lost during drying; dried hemlock in hay is apparently less poisonous than the fresh plant.

• POISONING Many people have died after eating hemlock, usually when it has been mistaken for other similar plants such as wild carrot or parsley. Even a small quantity can cause poisoning, with symptoms appearing in fifteen minutes to two hours. Initially there is burning and dryness of the mouth, followed by muscular weakness leading to paralysis that eventually affects the breathing. There may also be dilatation of pupils, vomiting, diarrhoea, convulsions and loss of consciousness.

Poisoning in animals is most likely in spring, when young leaves are eaten with other herbage, or on poor pasture, at any time of year, where the plant is dominant. All domestic animals can be poisoned by hemlock, although their susceptibility varies. Signs of poisoning appear within a few hours and include rapid breathing, excessive flow of saliva, difficulty in swallowing, diarrhoea, muscular weakness and trembling, sometimes with convulsions. The breath of poisoned animals may have the characteristic mousy smell of the plant. Adult pigs may appear blind, with swollen or closed eyes; later they may go into a deep sleep. The offspring of pregnant animals may have birth defects; limb and spinal deformities and cleft palate have been reported in piglets after the sows have eaten hemlock.

Because of the potentially severe nature of the poisoning, professional advice should be sought as soon as possible.

• NOTE The poisonous properties of hemlock have been known for over 2000 years and various preparations of the plant used deliberately to kill people. The most famous of these is Socrates, whose death in 399 BC has been attributed to his being made to drink an extract of hemlock (or possibly a related plant). Hemlock was referred to as 'a naughtie and dangerous herbe' in a herbal by Henry Lyte in 1578.

Giant Hogweed

Heracleum mantegazzianum (photo 80)

Since its introduction to Britain in the last century, giant hogweed has spread to many parts of the country and can now be seen beside rivers, along railways and on roadsides as well as in gardens and at the edges of fields. When fully grown it is an unmistakable, large plant often more than 3 m (10 ft) tall. The stems are about 5 cm (2 in) across and are strong, ridged, hollow and usually purple-spotted. The lower leaves can be 1 m (3 ft) long and are deeply lobed and toothed; the upper ones are smaller and the base of the leaf stalk is greatly inflated where it sheathes the stem. The flower heads (umbels) at the top of the plant are large and distinctive, up to 5 cm (20 in) across, and composed of 50–150 separate stalks (rays), each with a group of small white flowers at the top. The lateral umbels are smaller and usually composed mostly of male flowers.

• POISONOUS SUBSTANCES The sap of the plant contains furocoumarins, which, on contact, sensitize the skin to the ultraviolet rays in sunlight (photosensitization). All parts of the plant contain these substances, but it seems that soil conditions and climate influence their concentration. Their highest content has been found in spring, with a decrease in the following months.

• POISONING Injury to the skin results from exposure to sunlight after direct contact with the sap. This can happen either by touching the plant or by being sprayed with sap when cutting it down; such spray has been known to penetrate clothing. The circumstances under which skin damage usually occurs include accidentally brushing against the plant when walking, contact with the plant when cutting it down or digging it up and, in children, using various parts of the plant when playing. Reddening, stinging and irritation of the affected areas of skin occur within 24 hours, followed by the development of large, fluid-filled blisters that can be very painful. These usually subside quickly, but leave brown patches that can persist for several months.

Similar effects on the skin and in the mouth have occurred in ducklings, goats and sheep, but, in general, little is known about the effects of giant hogweed on animals as they do not usually touch or eat the plant.

If extensive areas of skin are affected or severe reactions occur, professional advice should be sought.

• NOTE Care should be taken not to allow this spectacular plant to grow in areas where children are likely to play. General control measures to reduce its spread in other areas have been advocated.

Hemlock Water Dropwort

Oenanthe crocata (photos 81 and 82)

Dead Men's Fingers

This plant grows in wet areas, not normally on chalky soil, and is scattered throughout Britain, but mainly in the south and west. The stems are up to 1·5 m (5 ft) tall and are hollow, grooved and slender, about 1 cm (⅓ in) across. The lower leaves, with stalks that sheathe the stem, may exceed 30 cm (12 in) in length. They are subdivided into leaflets with deeply divided lobes and bluntly toothed edges; the upper leaves have one or two leaflets, with narrower segments. The flower heads (umbels) are composed of domed groups of small white flowers, each group growing on a separate stalk (ray). The rays are of unequal length so that the flower head is not flat topped as in some other members of this family. The root tubers of hemlock water dropwort are characteristic, and it is from these that the alternative common name, dead men's fingers, is derived; below ground there is a bunch of white or yellowish-white, tapering tubers containing juice that becomes yellow when exposed to the air. Each tuber is up to 10 cm (4 in) long and 1-2 cm (⅓-¾ in) wide; they are reputed to have a sweetish taste.

● POISONOUS SUBSTANCE Oenanthetoxin, an unsaturated higher alcohol, is found in all parts of the plant, especially in the roots, where its concentration is highest in winter and early spring. The toxin remains active in the dried plant and after cooking.

● POISONING Hemlock water dropwort is one of the most poisonous plants in Britain; more than half of the cases of human poisoning are fatal. Most incidents arise from misidentification of the plant. Some recent ones have resulted from the current interest in collecting wild plants for food; the roots have been eaten raw, boiled, or added to soup. Symptoms develop within an hour or two and include nausea, excessive production of saliva, repeated vomiting, diarrhoea, profuse sweating, weakness of the legs and dilatation of the pupils; later there may be loss of consciousness with convulsions before death. Accidental splashing of sap in the eye of a laboratory worker led to symptoms of poisoning lasting for 12 hours.

Animals are also highly susceptible to hemlock water dropwort poisoning, which is most likely to occur when the roots are exposed during land drainage or ditch cleaning. The symptoms are much the same as in human poisoning, although cattle often die suddenly, without symptoms being seen.

Professional help should be sought urgently, because the stomach contents need to be removed and barbiturate drugs injected to control the convulsions.

● NOTE This plant is dangerously poisonous, even in small quantities. There are other *Oenanthe* species that cause similar, but less severe, poisoning.

URTICACEAE

The nettles in this family appear to be harmless when eaten, but the stinging sensation produced by contact with them is well known; the so-called dead nettles in the Labiatae family do not have this effect.

Stinging Nettle *Urtica dioica* (photo 83)

Stinging nettles are abundant throughout Britain in woods and hedges and on waste or neglected land. They have much-branched, tough, yellowish roots that spread through the ground and produce erect shoots in spring, often forming dense clumps. The plants grow up to 1 m (3 ft) tall; the stems are ridged or square and bear leaves in pairs. These are coarse, pointed, toothed at the edges and 4–7·5 cm (1½–3 in) long. The leaves and stems have numerous stiff stinging hairs. The flowers are small and packed together in spikes that are erect or drooping like tassels and uniformly green.

• POISONOUS SUBSTANCES For many years it was thought that formic acid was released when the hairs were touched, but histamine, acetylcholine and 5-hydroxytryptamine are now known to be involved in the stinging reaction.

• POISONING Nettles are occasionally eaten fresh in salads, cooked like spinach, or used to make a tea; no reports of poisoning following these practices have been found. It is by skin contact with the stinging hairs on the leaf and stem that nettles exert adverse effects. Initially there is a pricking sensation, rapidly followed by reddening, soreness and the development of raised, white patches; there is often considerable itching later. The symptoms usually subside within a few hours, but may persist for a day or two.

In general, animals are not affected by nettle stings, but in the USA there have been reports of hunting dogs that developed trembling, vomiting, difficult breathing and general weakness, following contact with large numbers of nettle plants; some dogs died.

VERBENACEAE

Members of the genus *Lantana* cause serious poisoning of livestock in parts of the world where they grow wild. In Britain, however, they are grown only as house or garden plants. Pigeon berry (*Duranta repens*), another member of this family cultivated here, is also poisonous (see list, page 109).

Lantana *Lantana* species (photo 84)

The common lantana or yellow sage (*Lantana camara*), and also *Lantana montevidensis*, a more delicate plant with a weeping habit, are the two most likely to be seen in this country, either in gardens or as glasshouse or house plants; no *Lantana* species grow wild in this country. *Lantana* species are small shrubs with pointed or oval leaves, 4–6 cm (1½–2½ in) long, having a rather coarse appearance; some leaves have scalloped edges. The flowers are produced most of the year. They grow closely packed together in flat or domed clusters and are shades of yellow, orange, pink or red, depending on the variety.

• POISONOUS SUBSTANCE The leaves and fruits contain lantadene A, a polycyclic triterpene. There are, however, some non-toxic varieties that do not contain this toxin. The green, unripe fruits ('berries') are especially toxic and are responsible for most cases of human poisoning.

• POISONING Young children have been poisoned, occasionally fatally, by eating the green berries; although these are less toxic when ripe, it is unwise to eat them at any stage. Signs of poisoning develop within a few hours: weakness, vomiting, diarrhoea, inability to stand, slow deep breathing and, usually, dilatation of pupils. In severe cases, where stomach contents have not been removed, unconsciousness, coma and death have also been reported.

Lantana poisoning is unlikely to occur in animals in Britain as here it is grown only as a garden plant, but in other countries, where the plant grows wild, cattle, sheep and goats are affected and there can be serious economic losses. Digestive-system disturbances, with constipation, occur initially. In severe cases there may be general weakness and staggering, mouth ulceration and blindness. Liver damage leads to jaundice and an abnormal response of unpigmented areas of skin to sunlight (photosensitization), with reddening, swelling, oozing of fluid, scab formation and cracking. Dogs have also been affected; they appear lethargic, with digestive-system disturbances, including vomiting.

Professional help is needed as the plant material must be removed from the stomach. Charcoal, given by mouth, has been successful in treating sheep.

Crop plants

Although it is an apparent contradiction, there are certain crops grown specifically for human or animal food that can, under certain conditions, be harmful to eat. It must be emphasized that these are not poisonous plants in the generally accepted sense and it is only when they are used inappropriately that adverse effects occur. The main plants in this category belong to four families: Chenopodiaceae including various types of beet; Cruciferae, including kale, rape and turnips; Gramineae including grasses and cereal crops; and Leguminosae, including clover and beans.

The tops of sugar beet, and the roots of these and other beet croops are a valuable source of winter feed for livestock. There are, however, certain toxic conditions that may develop if they are fed incorrectly. The two most important of these are nitrate-nitrite and oxalate poisoning. There may also be digestive-system disturbances, and sugar beet tops can taint the milk of cows.

The hot taste common to members of the Cruciferae family is due to the presence of a substance called mustard oil, an isothiocyanate, which can cause enlargement of the thyroid gland (goitre). They also contain a substance (S-methyl cysteine sulphoxide, usually abbreviated to SMCO) that can cause anaemia. Other effects reported in various animal species, including poultry, are blindness, digestive-system disturbances, breathing difficulties, leg weakness, decreased egg production and a taint in eggs and meat. All of these effects occur only if an excess of cruciferous plants are fed.

Although grasses and grain are excellent as animal feeds and are the main ingredients of many feed mixes, there are certain diseases associated with their use. A change to good pasture in autumn can result in cattle eating too much herbage containing tryptophan, which causes a sudden and sometimes fatal illness, called fog fever, that affects breathing. Too much grain without adequate roughage can cause digestive-system disturbances, and grain contaminated by fungi can cause illness due to the production of mycotoxins (page 111).

In the Leguminosae family, lupins grown as fodder crops sometimes contain alkaloids that can cause staggering, convulsions, and deformity of the young. Lupin varieties that do not contain these alkaloids are now being produced. Another disease, lupinosis, characterized by poor growth and jaundice due to liver damage, is caused by fungi often found on the plants. Clover and lucerne contain substances (oestrogens) that can have an adverse effect on the reproductive performance of animals. The many types of beans used extensively as human food, especially by vegetarians, can also cause poisoning if eaten raw or inadequately cooked. The main effects (nausea, vomiting, diarrhoea, low body temperature and rapid heart rate) are due to the presence of simple proteins, called lectins. It is essential to apply sufficient heat over an adequate period of cooking time to destroy them. Cooking in a slow cooker does not destroy them, as the temperature is too low, but boiling for at least 20 minutes, or cooking in a pressure cooker ensures that the lectins are denatured, after which the beans are completely safe to eat.

It should be emphasized that all of the animal and human foods in this category are excellent nutritionally and recommended, provided that they are used only in the correct way (as explained in agricultural, veterinary or cookery books).

Other poisonous plants
An annotated list

This list includes plants of low or doubtful toxicity, plants that are not common in Britain and plants that occur here but have caused poisoning only in other countries.

It cannot be assumed that related species or varieties are necessarily poisonous or harmless, as variations in toxicity exist even among closely related plants.

The plants are arranged in alphabetical order of families, so that similar plants are grouped together. Within the families they are arranged alphabetically by their scientific (Latin) names.

Plant	Type of plant and effects
ACERACEAE	
Red Maple *Acer rubrum*	Garden and parkland tree. Horses eating the leaves have become anaemic; some have died.
AMARYLLIDACEAE	
Kaffir Lily *Clivia miniata*	House plant. Similar to daffodil poisoning (page 20).
Cape Lily *Crinum* species	Garden plants. Similar to daffodil poisoning (page 20).
Snowdrop *Galanthus nivalis*	Garden plant, sometimes wild. Similar to daffodil poisoning (page 20).
Blood Lily *Haemanthus* species	House plants. Similar to daffodil poisoning (page 20).
Amaryllis *Hippeastrum* species	House plants. Mild digestive-system disturbances if many bulbs eaten. Photo 2.
Snowflake *Leucojum* species	Garden plants. Similar to daffodil poisoning (page 20).
Nerines including **Guernsey Lily** *Nerine* species	Garden plants. Similar to daffodil poisoning (page 20).

Plant	Type of plant and effects
ANACARDIACEAE	
Sumac *Rhus typhina*	Garden tree. Raw fruits and leaves can cause mild digestive-system disturbances. Not to be confused with poison sumac (*Toxicodendron vernix*), found in Britain only in botanical gardens.
APOCYNACEAE	
Allamanda *Allamanda* species	House plants. Can cause severe diarrhoea. Sap irritant to skin.
Madagascar Periwinkle *Catharanthus roseus* (sometimes called *Vinca rosea*)	House plant. Contains toxic alkaloids.
Dipladenia *Dipladenia* species	House plants. Similar to *Allamanda* poisoning (above).
ARACEAE	
Elephant's Ear *Alocasia* species	House plants. Similar to *Dieffenbachia* poisoning (page 25) but less severe.
Jack in the Pulpit *Arisaema* species	House plants. Similar to *Dieffenbachia* poisoning (page 25) but less severe.
Bog Arum *Calla palustris*	Aquatic plant. Similar to wild arum poisoning (page 23).
Elephant's Ear *Colocasia* species	House plants. Similar to *Dieffenbachia* poisoning (page 25) but less severe.
Devil's Ivy *Epipremnum pinnatum* (sometimes called *Epipremnum aureum,* *Pothos aureus,* *Rhaphidophora aurea* or *Scindapsus aureus*)	House plant. Similar to *Dieffenbachia* poisoning (page 25) but less severe.
Syngonium *Syngonium* species (sometimes called *Nephthytis*).	House plants. Similar to *Dieffenbachia* poisoning (page 25) but less severe.

Plant	Type of plant and effects
ARISTOLOCHIACEAE	
Birthwort *Aristolochia* species	Garden plants, sometimes wild. Particularly poisonous to horses, causing copious urination, rapid heart rate, paralysis and coma.
ASCLEPIADACEAE	
Milkweed *Asclepias* species	Garden plants. Contain glycosides that affect the heart. Poisoning not reported in Britain.
BEGONIACEAE	
Begonia *Begonia* species	House and garden plants. Often suspected, but generally regarded as not poisonous.
BERBERIDACEAE	
Mahonia *Mahonia* species	Garden shrubs. Berries harmless, other parts may contain berberine (page 29).
CACTACEAE	
Peyote *Lophophora williamsii*	Cactus. Has hallucinogenic properties, also causes nausea, vomiting, shivering and panic.
CAMPANULACEAE	
Lobelia *Lobelia* species	Garden plants. Human poisoning unlikely, but sap can cause skin reactions. Poisoning rare in animals, but similar to deadly nightshade (page 76).
CAPRIFOLIACEAE	
Honeysuckle *Lonicera* species	Garden and wild plants. Berries (various colours) harmless or of very low toxicity.

Plant	Type of plant and effects
Guelder Rose, **Wayfaring Tree** and others *Viburnum* species	Garden and wild plants. Unripe berries or a large number of ripe berries (red or black) can cause mild vomiting and diarrhoea.

CARYOPHYLLACEAE

Plant	Type of plant and effects
Corn Cockle *Agrostemma githago*	Garden and wild plant. Formerly common in cereal crops, now rare in Britain. Seeds contain saponins that can cause digestive-system disturbances.
Sandwort *Arenaria* species	Garden and wild plants. Poisoning unlikely but contain saponins that could cause digestive-system disturbances.
Soapwort *Saponaria* species	Garden and wild plants. Contain saponins that can cause mild digestive-system disturbances.
Chickweed *Stellaria* species	Wild plants. Contain saponins that can cause mild digestive-system disturbances if eaten in large amounts.

COMMELINACEAE

Plant	Type of plant and effects
Wandering Jew *Tradescantia* species	House plants. Skin contact can result in reddening and blistering.

COMPOSITAE

Plant	Type of plant and effects
Greater Burdock *Arctium lappa*	Wild plant. The small hooks on the seed head can cause soreness and ulceration of the mouth, and skin damage.
Wormwood *Artemesia absinthium*	Garden and wild plant. Eating large amounts has caused poisoning in animals in other countries. May taint milk.
Mugwort *Artemisia vulgaris*	Wild plants. Eating large amounts has caused digestive-system disturbances and even death of cattle in other countries.

Plant	Type of plant and effects
Thistle *Carduus* species	Garden and wild plants. Can accumulate toxic amounts of nitrates but no reports of poisoning in Britain.
Yellow Star Thistle, St. Barnaby's Thistle *Centaurea solstitialis*	Wild plant. Causes a severe nervous-system disorder of horses in countries where it is plentiful. No reports of poisoning in Britain.
Chrysanthemum *Chrysanthemum* species	Garden and wild plants. Can cause allergic skin reactions and symptoms like hay fever. Herbal remedies containing it have caused poisoning.
Chicory *Cichorium intybus*	Garden and wild plants. The roots have caused diarrhoea, paralysis and death of cattle.
Thistle *Cirsium* species	Garden and wild plants. Can accumulate toxic amounts of nitrates but no reports of poisoning in Britain.
Leopard's Bane *Doronicum* species	Garden and wild plants. Poisoning rare but reported in pigs.
Sunflower *Helianthus* species	Crop and garden plants. Young plants have caused nitrate poisoning of cattle.
Ploughman's Spikenard *Inula conyza*	Wild plant. Has caused digestive-system disturbances and death of cattle and sheep in other countries.
Groundsel *Senecio vulgaris*	Wild plant. Contains alkaloids similar to those in ragwort (page 36). Generally not growing in sufficient quantities to cause poisoning.
Milk Thistle *Silybum marianum*	Garden and wild plants. Contains nitrates that have caused poisoning of cattle in other countries.
Golden Rod *Solidago* species	Garden plants, occasionally growing wild. Can accumulate toxic amounts of nitrates, but poisoning unlikely in Britain.
Cocklebur *Xanthium strumarium*	Wild plant. Has caused digestive- and nervous-system disturbances and death of farm animals in other countries.

Plant	Type of plant and effects
CONVOLVULACEAE	
Dodder *Cuscuta* species	Wild parasitic plants. Can cause digestive-system disturbances. Horses are especially susceptible. Unlikely to be eaten in any appreciable quantity in Britain.
CORNACEAE	
Spotted Laurel *Aucuba japonica*	Garden shrub. Fruits slightly poisonous, causing diarrhoea.
Dogwood *Cornus* species	Garden and wild plants. Fruits slightly poisonous, causing diarrhoea. Leaves can cause skin irritation.
CRASSULACEAE	
Crassula *Crassula* species	Garden and wild plants. Similar to *Sedum spectabile* poisoning (below).
Stonecrop *Sedum acre*	Garden and wild plant. Similar to *Sedum spectabile* poisoning (below).
Sedum *Sedum spectabile*	Garden plant. Sap can cause irritation and blistering of skin. Unlikely to be eaten by animals, but has caused mild poisoning of pigs.
CRUCIFERAE	
Shepherd's Purse *Capsella bursa-pastoris*	Wild plant. Can taint milk.
Swine Cress *Coronopus* species	Wild plant. Toxicity doubtful, but can taint milk.
Wild Radish *Raphanus raphanistrum*	Wild plant. Similar to charlock poisoning (below). Hot-tasting white root harmless in small amounts.
Charlock *Sinapis arvensis*	Wild plant. Causes digestive-system disturbances if large quantities eaten at seeding stage.

Plant	Type of plant and effects
CUPRESSACEAE	
Juniper *Juniperus* species	Garden and wild plants. Similar to cypress poisoning (page 40); also cause digestive-system disturbances.
Chinese, Northern **White** and **Western** **Red Cedar** *Thuja* species	Garden and parkland trees or hedges. Unlikely to be eaten but can cause severe digestive-system disturbances, with liver and kidney damage.
CYPERACEAE	
Sedge *Carex* species	Garden and wild plants. Contain glycosides that can cause cyanide poisoning (see laurel, page 73).
ERICACEAE	
Bog Rosemary, Marsh **Andromeda** *Andromeda polifolia*	Garden and wild plant. Toxicity doubtful. Said to be similar to rhododendron poisoning but less severe (page 45).
Calico Bush, Mountain **Laurel** and others *Kalmia* species	Garden shrubs, Similar to rhododendron poisoning (page 45); toxicity variable.
Menziesia *Menziesia* species	Garden shrubs. Similar to rhododendron poisoning (page 45).
EUPHORBIACEAE	
Croton *Codiaeum* species	House plants. Similar to spurge poisoning (page 47), but can be more severe. Poisoning not reported in Britain. Photo 33.
Caper Spurge *Euphorbia lathyrus*	Garden plant; sometimes wild. Similar to petty and sun spurge poisoning (page 47). Seed pods sometimes mistaken for edible capers.
Zig-Zag Plant *Pedilanthus tithymaloides*	House plant. Similar to spurge poisoning (page 47), but less severe.

Plant	Type of plant and effects
African Milkbush *Synadenium grantii*	House plant. Similar to spurge poisoning (page 47).
FUMARIACEAE **Dutchman's Breeches,** **Bleeding Heart** *Dicentra* species	Garden plants. Can cause trembling, staggering and convulsions. Poisoning rare.
GERANIACEAE **Storksbill** *Erodium* species	Garden and wild plants. Have produced skin reactions (photosensitization) in cattle and sheep in other countries.
HYDRANGEACEAE **Hydrangea** *Hydrangea* species	Garden plants. If large amounts eaten can cause cyanide poisoning (see laurel, page 73)
IRIDACEAE **Gladiolus** *Gladiolus* species	Garden plants. Eating the corms has caused digestive-system disturbances.
JUNCACEAE **Rush** *Juncus* species	Garden and wild plants. Have caused digestive-system disturbances and temporary blindness of cattle. Some species can cause cyanide poisoning (see laurel, page 73).
JUNCAGINACEAE **Arrow Grass** *Triglochin* species	Wild plants. Have caused cyanide poisoning (see laurel, page 73) of livestock but no reports in Britain.

Plant	Type of plant and effects
LABIATAE	
Hemp Nettle *Galeopsis* species	Wild plants. Seeds have caused death of horses and pigs in Russia.
Ground Ivy *Glechoma hederacea*	Garden and wild plant. Has caused breathing difficulties and death of horses and cattle in eastern Europe.
Henbit, Dead Nettle *Lamium* species	Garden and wild plants. Have poisoned livestock. No recent reports.
Mint *Mentha* species	Garden and wild plants. Poisoning rare. Increased urine production and nervous-system damage. Sap can cause skin irritation and blistering.
LEGUMINOSAE	
Milk Vetch *Astragalus* species	Garden and wild plants. Some species harmless, others poisonous. Severe poisoning of livestock in USA; no reports of poisoning in Britain.
Bird of Paradise *Caesalpinia gilliesii*	Garden shrub. Leaves and seeds cause vomiting and diarrhoea. Other *Caesalpinia* species (including some also called *Poinciana*) are poisonous.
Crown Vetch *Coronilla varia*	Garden and wild plant. Apparently not toxic to cattle, sheep and goats. Has caused reduced growth rate, paralysis and death of pigs in other countries.
Broom *Cytisus scoparius*	Wild plant. Very large quantities can affect the heart and nervous system.
Goat's Rue, French Honeysuckle *Galega officinalis*	Garden plant, sometimes wild. Can cause breathing difficulties, loss of muscular coordination, convulsions and death of sheep, occasionally cattle.
Sweet Pea *Lathyrus odoratus*	Garden plant. Eating a large number of seeds can cause temporary paralysis.
Birdsfoot Trefoil *Lotus corniculatus*	Wild plant. Has caused cyanide poisoning (see laurel, page 73) in other countries.

101

Plant	Type of plant and effects
Sweet Clover *Melilotus* species	Fodder crop. Has caused severe haemorrhages, mainly in cattle, in other countries. Can taint milk.
False Acacia *Robinia pseudoacacia*	Garden tree, sometimes wild. Has caused digestive-system disturbances and coma of animals in other countries.
Spanish Broom *Spartium junceum*	Garden plant. Similar to broom poisoning (above).
Vetch *Vicia* species	Wild plants. Some can cause cyanide poisoning (see laurel, page 73). No reports of poisoning in Britain.
Wisteria *Wisteria* species	Garden plants. All parts poisonous. Pods or a few seeds have caused digestive-system disturbances, with repeated vomiting.

LILIACEAE

Aloe *Aloe* species	House plants. Sap contains an anthraquinone glycoside that is purgative; sometimes causes red urine.
Asparagus *Asparagus* species	House plants and cultivated crop. Red berries slightly poisonous. Touching young shoots can cause dermatitis.
Spider Plant *Chlorophytum* species	House and garden plants. Similar to tulip poisoning (below).
Fritillary *Fritillaria* species	Garden plants, very occasionally wild. Bulbs have produced vomiting and effects on the heart in children and dogs.
Glory Lily *Gloriosa superba*	House plant. Contains the alkaloid colchicine. Similar to autumn crocus poisoning (page 57).
Hyacinth *Hyacinthus* species	Garden and house plants. Bulbs have caused severe diarrhoea and death in cattle. Sap can cause dermatitis.
Star of Bethlehem *Ornithogalum umbellatum*	Garden plant. Flowers and bulbs have produced digestive-system disturbances.

102

Plant	Type of plant and effects
Chincherinchee *Ornithogalum thyrsoides*	House plant and cut flowers. Can produce severe digestive-system disturbances.
Squill, Scilla *Scilla* species	Garden and wild plants. Similar to bluebell poisoning (page 59).
Tulip *Tulipa* species	Garden plants. Bulbs mistaken for onions have caused vomiting and weakness.

LOGANIACEAE

Yellow Jasmine *Gelsemium sempervirens*	Garden plant. All parts, but particularly nectar, poisonous. Causes muscular weakness and breathing difficulty; sometimes fatal. No reports of poisoning in Britain.

MALVACEAE

Mallow *Malva* species	Garden and wild plants. Have caused loss of coordination and death, particularly of sheep in Australia.

MELIACEAE

Chinaberry *Melia azedarach*	Garden tree. All parts poisonous, causing vomiting, diarrhoea, breathing difficulties; if severe, paralysis and death. No reports of poisoning in Britain.

MORACEAE

Rubber Plant *Ficus elastica*	House plant. The sap (latex) has caused vomiting and diarrhoea.

NYCTAGINACEAE

Four o'clock Plant *Mirabilis jalapa*	Garden plant. Seeds and roots can cause digestive-system disturbances.

Plant	Type of plant and effects
OROBANCHACEAE	
Broomrape *Orobanche* species	Wild parasitic plants. Rarely eaten by animals but have caused digestive-system disturbances.
OXALIDACEAE	
Wood Sorrel *Oxalis acetosella*	Wild plant. Contains oxalates (page 68) and has caused poisoning in animals in other countries.
PAEONIACEAE	
Peony *Paeonia* species	Garden plants. Of doubtful toxicity but may cause mild digestive-system disturbances.
PAPAVERACEAE	
Prickly Poppy *Argemone* species	Garden plants. Contain toxic alkaloids that can affect the nervous system.
Yellow Horned Poppy *Glaucium flavum*	Garden and wild plant. Contains poisonous alkaloids, but no record of poisoning in Britain.
Long-headed Poppy *Papaver dubium*	Wild plant. has caused poisoning of animals in other countries.
Iceland Poppy *Papaver nudicaule*	Garden plant. Similar to field poppy poisoning (page 65).
PINACEAE	
Western Yellow Pine *Pinus ponderosa*	Garden tree. Can cause abortion in late pregnancy in cattle.
POLYGONACEAE	
Buckwheat *Fagopyrum esculentum*	Cultivated crop. Causes skin sensitivity to light (photosensitization) in animals (see St. John's wort, page 53).

Plant	Type of plant and effects
Knotgrass, Snakeroot and others *Polygonum* species	Garden and wild plants. Can cause digestive-system disturbances. No record of poisoning in Britain. Sap irritant to skin.
Common Sorrel *Rumex acetosa*	Wild plant. Contains oxalates (page 68), which can cause kidney damage and death of animals.
Sheep's Sorrel *Rumex acetosella*	Wild plant. Similar to common sorrel poisoning (above).

PRIMULACEAE

Scarlet Pimpernel *Anagallis arvensis*	Wild plant. Toxicity varies. Contains saponins that have caused digestive-system and kidney disturbances in animals. Can cause dermatitis.
Cyclamen *Cyclamen* species	Garden and house plants, occasionally wild. Corms cause digestive-system disturbances, and sometimes convulsions, reddish coloration of urine, irregular heart beat, and death. No recent reports.
Primula *Primula* species	Garden, wild and house plants. Skin contact with some species, particularly *Primula obconica,* can cause severe dermatitis. If eaten, digestive-system disturbances can result.

RANUNCULACEAE

Baneberry *Actaea* species	Garden and wild plants. Reputed to cause digestive-system disturbances and signs of confusion.
Pheasant's Eye *Adonis annua*	Garden plant, occasionally wild. Contains glycosides, which affect the heart, and possibly protoanemonin. No reports of poisoning in Britain.
Columbine *Aquilegia* species	Garden and wild plants. Contain alkaloids similar to those in monkshood (page 69). No reports of poisoning in Britain.

Plant	Type of plant and effects
Marsh Marigold, Kingcup *Caltha palustris*	Wild plant. Similar to buttercup poisoning (page 71). Photo 61.
Delphinium, Larkspur *Delphinium* species	Garden plants. Similar to monkshood poisoning (page 69).
Stinking Hellebore *Helleborus foetidus*	Garden plant, occasionally wild. See Christmas rose (below).
Christmas Rose, Easter Rose *Helleborus niger*	Garden plant. Can cause excessive flow of saliva, digestive-system disturbances, and irregular heart beat. Poisoning rare.
Green Hellebore *Helleborus viridis*	Garden plant, occasionally wild. See Christmas rose (above).
Meadow Rue *Thalictrum* species	Garden and wild plants. Contain protoanemonin. Similar to buttercup poisoning (page 71). No record of poisoning in Britain.
Globe Flower *Trollius* species	Garden and wild plants. Contain protoanemonin. Similar to buttercup poisoning (page 71). No record of poisoning in Britain.

ROSACEAE

Ornamental Quince *Chaenomeles* species	Garden shrubs or trees. Seeds and leaves contain small amounts of glycosides that can cause cyanide poisoning (see laurel, page 73).
Cotoneaster *Cotoneaster* species	Garden shrubs, occasionally wild. All parts, including berries, contain variable amounts of glycosides that could cause cyanide poisoning (see laurel, page 73). Generally of very low toxicity and only mild digestive-system disturbances reported.
Hawthorn *Crataegus* species	Garden and wild shrubs or trees. Can cause dark coloration of urine in cattle and a fall in milk yield.

Plant	Type of plant and effects
Quince *Cydonia oblonga*	Garden tree. See apple (below).
Apple *Malus* species	Garden and orchard trees. Eating a large number of pips can cause cyanide poisoning (see laurel, page 73). Leaves may be toxic and unripe fruits can cause stomach pains.
Almond *Prunus dulcis* (sometimes called *Amygdalus communis*)	Garden tree. Bitter almonds (not generally available in Britain) can cause cyanide poisoning (see laurel, page 73).
Firethorn *Pyracantha* species	Garden plants. See cotoneaster (above).
Pear *Pyrus* species	Garden and orchard trees. Similar to apple (above) but apparently less toxic.
Rowan or **Mountain** **Ash** and others *Sorbus* species	Garden and wild trees. Eating a large number of berries, especially when unripe, can cause mild digestive-system disturbances.

RUSCACEAE

Butcher's Broom *Ruscus aculeatus*	Garden plant, occasionally wild. Berries can cause mild digestive-system disturbances. Poisoning unlikely.

SALICACEAE

Willow *Salix* species	Garden and wild plants. Human poisoning has occurred with severe abdominal pain after eating the leaves, but poisoning unlikely.

SCROPHULARIACEAE

Toadflax *Linaria* species	Garden and wild plants. Said to cause cyanide poisoning (see laurel, page 73). Not recorded recently.

107

Plant	Type of plant and effects
Cow Wheat *Melampyrum* species	Wild plants. See toadflax poisoning (above).
Lousewort *Pedicularis sylvatica*	Wild plant. See toadflax poisoning (above).

SOLANACEAE

Plant	Type of plant and effects
Jessamine *Cestrum* species	Garden and house plants. Similar to deadly nightshade poisoning (page 76) but less severe.
Tomato *Lycopersicon lycopersicum*	Cultivated crop. The foliage has caused poisoning of pigs.
Duke of Argyll's Tea Plant *Lycium chinense*	Garden shrub, occasionally wild. Said to contain alkaloids similar to those of deadly nightshade (page 76), but is much less poisonous.
Apple of Peru, Poison Berry *Nicandra physalodes*	Garden plant. Similar to Chinese lantern poisoning (below).
Tobacco *Nicotiana tabacum*	Cultivated crop. Eating the leaves has caused digestive-system disturbances and death of pigs. Pregnant animals have produced malformed young.
Chinese or **Japanese Lantern** *Physalis alkekengi*	Garden plant. Unripe berries have caused digestive-system disturbances in children; apparently harmless when ripe.
Chalice Vine, Trumpet Flower *Solandra* species	Garden plants. Similar to black nightshade poisoning (page 80).
Apple of Sodom *Solanum sodomeum*	Garden plant. Similar to Christmas cherry poisoning (page 79).

TRILLIACEAE

Plant	Type of plant and effects
Herb Paris *Paris quadrifolia*	Garden and wild plant. The blue-black berries can cause vomiting, stomach ache and diarrhoea.

Plant	Type of plant and effects
UMBELLIFERAE	
Fool's Parsley *Aethusa cynapium*	Wild plant. Similar to hemlock poisoning (page 86) but less severe.
Cow Parsley *Anthriscus sylvestris*	Wild plant. Toxicity doubtful. Said to cause poisoning similar to hemlock (page 86) but less severe.
Celery *Apium graveolens*	Crop and wild plants. Contact with the plants and subsequent exposure to sunlight can cause skin damage (photosensitization). Fungi present may also cause or enhance this effect.
Lesser Water Parsnip *Berula erecta*	Wild plant. Said to be similar to greater water parsnip poisoning (below). No record of poisoning in Britain.
Rough Chervil *Chaerophyllum temulentum*	Wild plant. Similar to hemlock poisoning (page 86) but less severe.
Hogweed, Cow Parsnip *Heracleum sphondylium*	Wild plant. Similar to effects of giant hogweed (page 87), but less severe.
Parsnip and **Wild Parsnip** *Pastinaca sativa*	Crop and wild plants. Skin contact with sap and subsequent exposure to sunlight (photosensitization) can have effects similar to those of giant hogweed (page 87).
Greater Water Parsnip *Sium latifolium*	Wild plants. Said to cause digestive-system disturbances, sleepiness and occasionally death. Plant rare and no reports of poisoning in Britain.
VERBENACEAE	
Pigeon Berry *Duranta repens*	Garden shrub often used for hedging. Berries contain a saponin, said to cause sleepiness, swelling of lips and eyelids, increase in body temperature, digestive-system disturbances and convulsions. Poisoning rare.

Plant	Type of plant and effects
VITACEAE	
Virginia Creeper *Parthenocissus* *quinquefolia*	Garden plant often on walls. Berries and leaves contain oxalates (page 68), which can cause digestive-system disturbances, sleepiness and some loss of consciousness. Poisoning rare.

Colour Illustrations

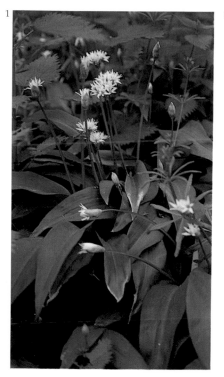

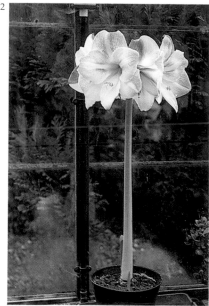

2 Amaryllis *(Hippeastrum species)*
HCB

1 Ramsons *(Allium ursinum)*
HCB

3 Daffodil *(Narcissus* species)
HCB

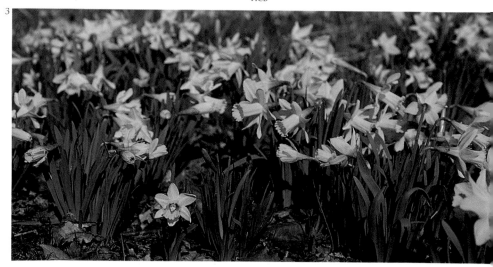

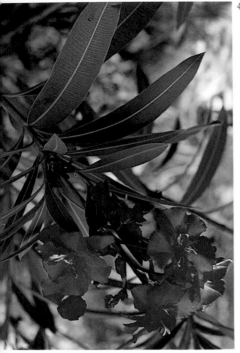

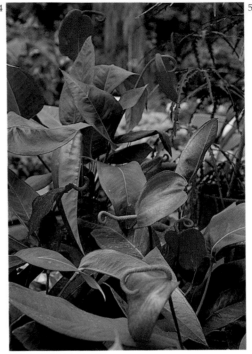

4   Oleander *(Nerium oleander)*
HCB

5   Flamingo Flower
(Anthurium species*)*
HCB

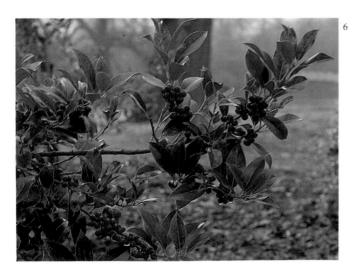

6   Holly *(Ilex aquifolium)*
SB

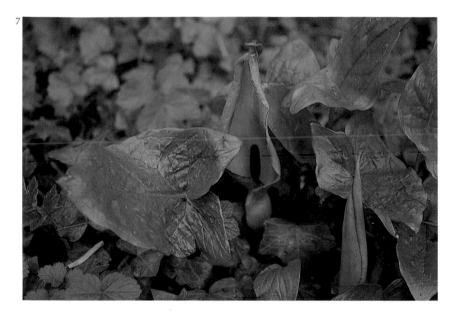

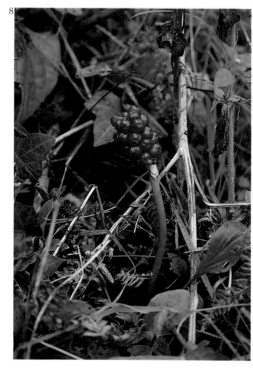

7   Cuckoo Pint *(Arum maculatum)*
     HCB

8   Cuckoo Pint *(Arum maculatum)*
     HCB

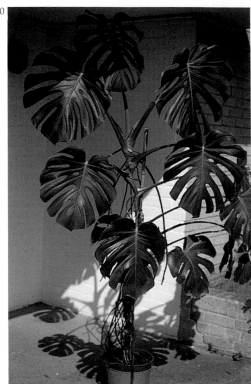

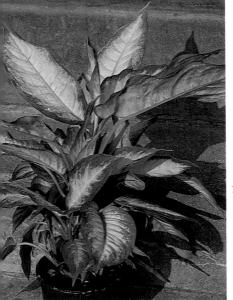

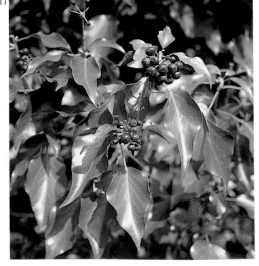

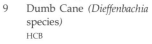

9   Dumb Cane *(Dieffenbachia* species*)*
HCB

10   Cheese Plant *(Monstera deliciosa)*
HCB

11   Ivy *(Hedera helix)*
HCB

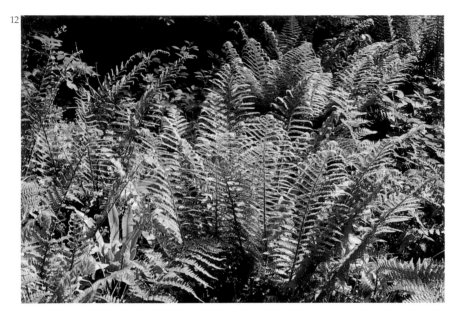

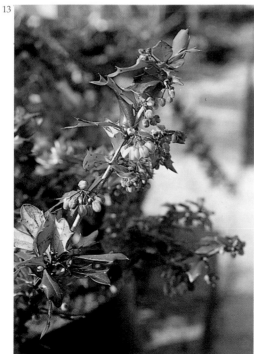

12 Male Fern *(Dryopteris*
    species*)*
    SB

13 Barberry *(Berberis* species*)*
    HCB

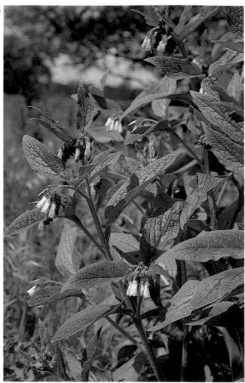

14 Comfrey *(Symphytum officinale)*
HCB

15 Purple Viper's Bugloss *(Echium plantagineum)*
HCB

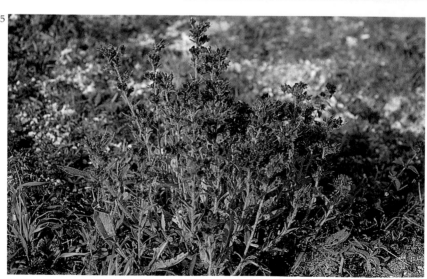

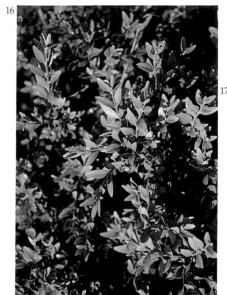

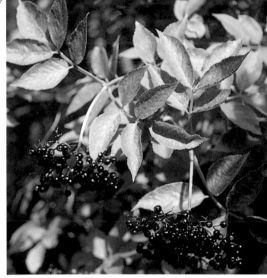

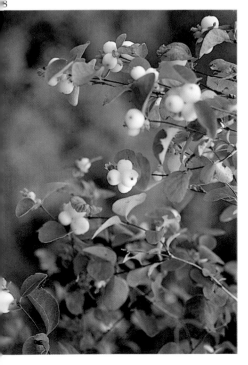

16 Box *(Buxus sempervirens)*
HCB

17 Elder *(Sambucus nigra)*
HCB

18 Snowberry *(Symphoricarpos
rivularis)*
HCB

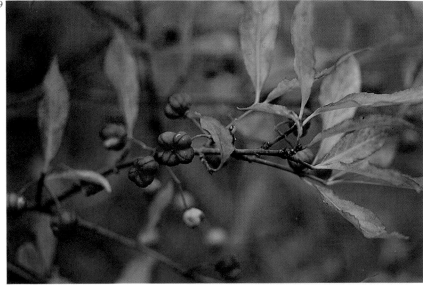

19   Spindle *(Euonymus europaeus)*
HCB

20   Fat Hen *(Chenopodium album)*
HCB

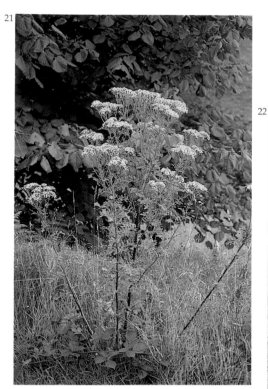

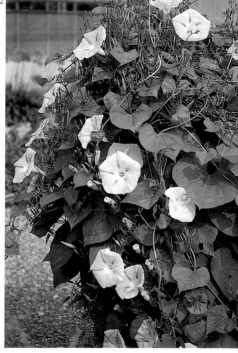

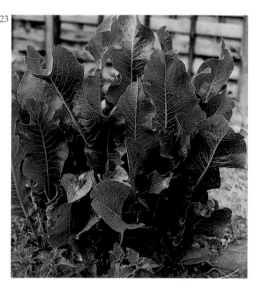

21 Ragwort *(Senecio jacobaea)*
HCB

22 Morning Glory *(Ipomoea
species)*
HCB

23 Horse Radish *(Armoracia
rusticana)*
HCB

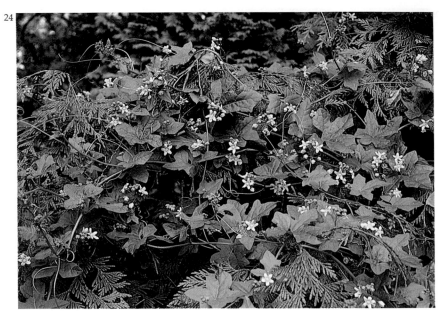

24   White Bryony *(Bryonia dioica)*
HCB

25   White Bryony *(Bryonia dioica)*
HCB

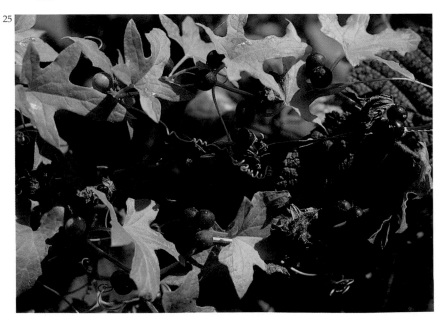

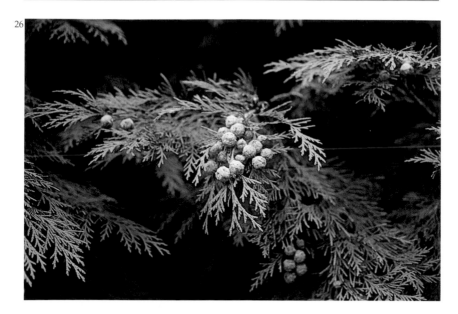

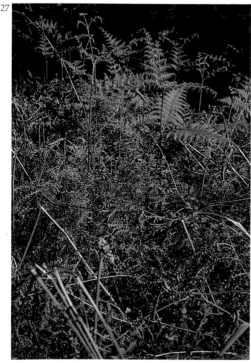

26 Cypress *(Cupressus species)*
HCB

27 Bracken *(Pteridium aquilinum)*
HCB

28

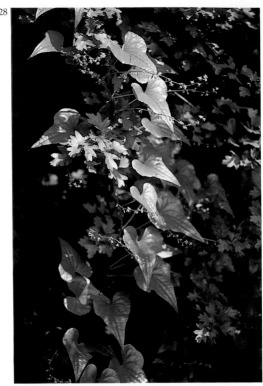

28   Black Bryony *(Tamus communis)*
HCB

29   Black Bryony *(Tamus communis)*
HCB

29

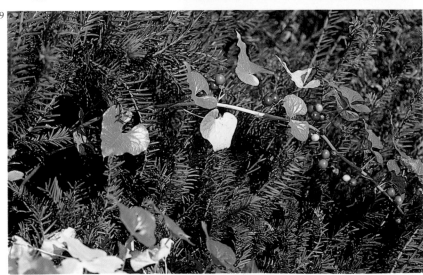

30 Horsetail *(Equisetum species)*
HCB

31 Pieris *(Pieris* species*)*
HCB

32

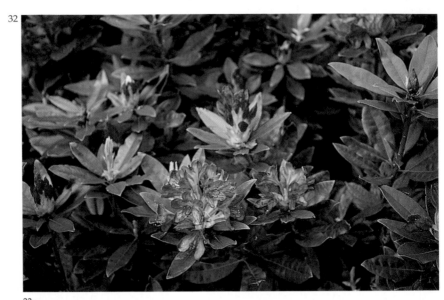

33

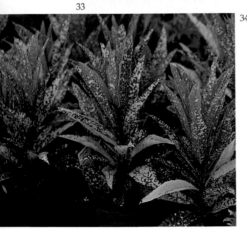

34

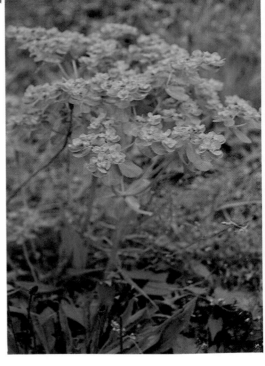

32 Rhododendron
    (Rhododendron ponticum)
    HCB

33 Croton *(Codiaeum* species*)*
    HCB

34 Sun Spurge *(Euphorbia
    helioscopia)*
    HCB

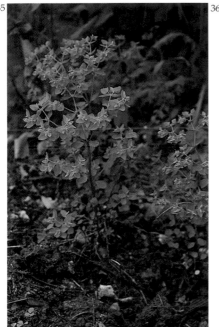

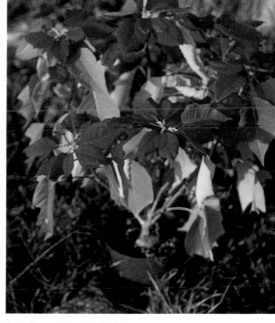

35 Petty Spurge *(Euphorbia peplus)*
HCB

36 Poinsettia *(Euphorbia pulcherrima)*
HCB

37 Dog's Mercury *(Mercurialis perennis)*
HCB

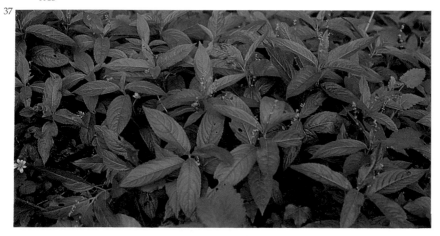

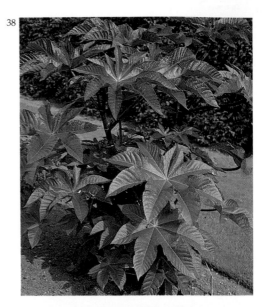

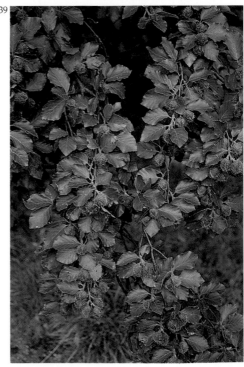

38 Castor Oil Plant *(Ricinus communis)*
    HCB

39 Beech *(Fagus sylvatica)*
    HCB

40
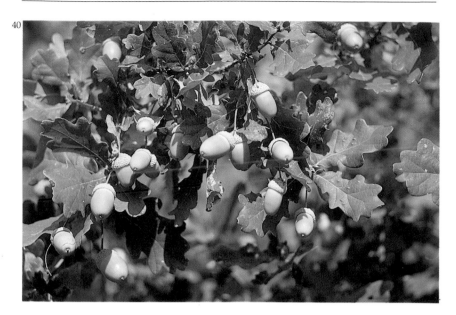

40   Oak *(Quercus pedunculata)*
HCB

41   Horse Chestnut *(Aesculus hippocastanum)*
HCB

41
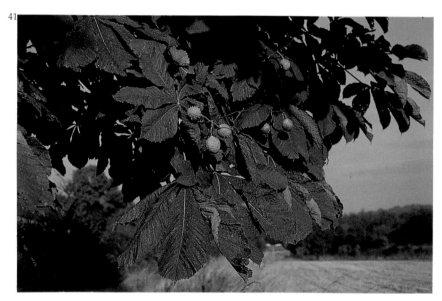

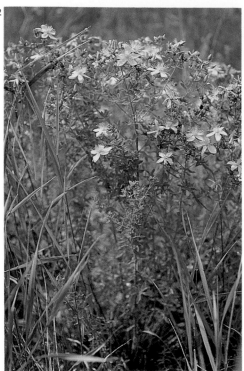

42   St John's Wort *(Hypericum perforatum)*
     HCB

43   Yellow Flag *(Iris pseudacorus)*
     HCB

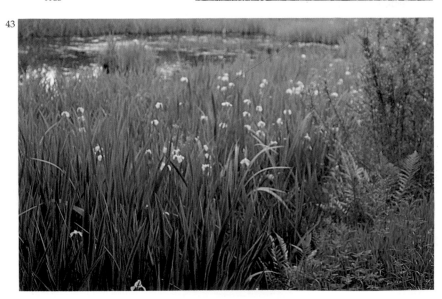

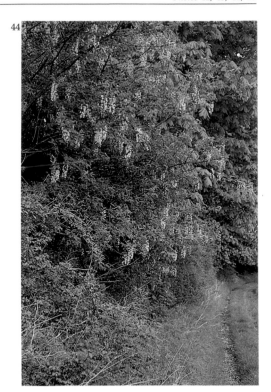

44 Laburnum *(Laburnum anagyroides)*
HCB

45 Laburnum *(Laburnum unagyroides)*
HCB

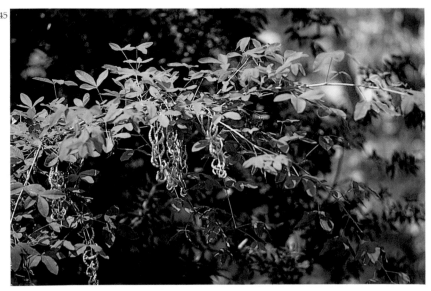

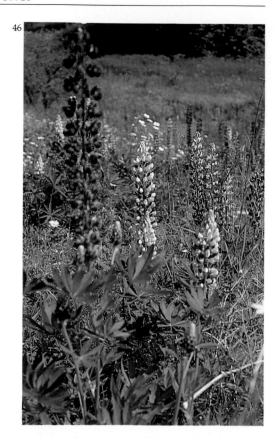

46   Lupin *(Lupinus* species)
HCB

47   Autumn Crocus
(Colchicum autumnale)
HCB

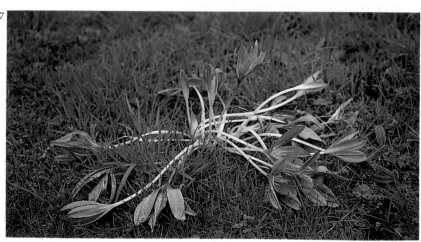

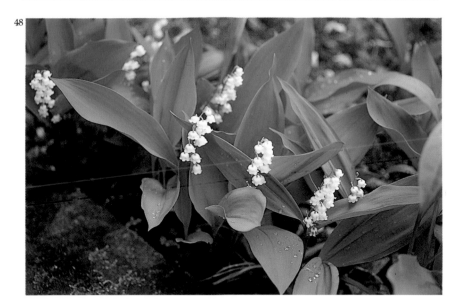

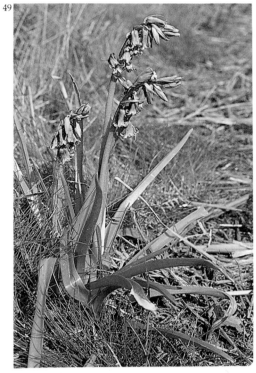

48 Lily of the Valley
  (Convallaria majalis)
  HCB

49 Bluebell *(Hyacinthoides*
  non-scripta)
  SB

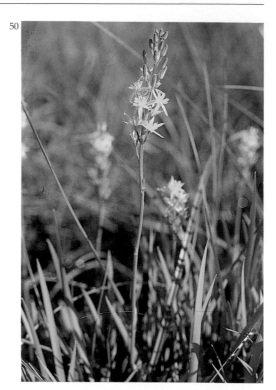

50 Bog Asphodel *(Narthecium ossifragum)*
HCB

51 Solomon's Seal *(Polygonatum multiflorum)*
HCB

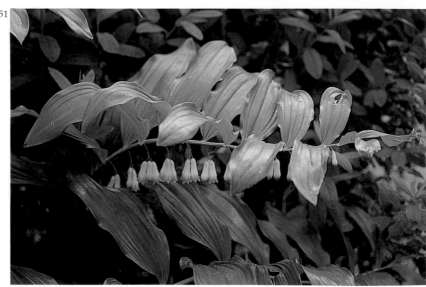

52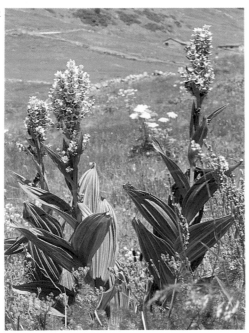

52 False Hellebore *(Veratrum species)*
SB

53 Mistletoe *(Viscum album)*
A-Z

53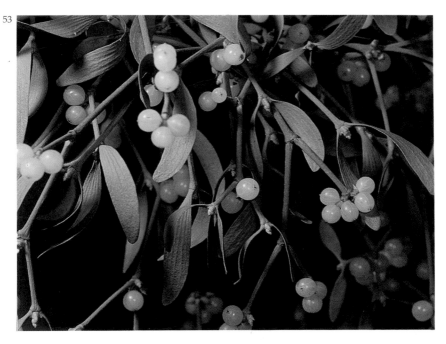

54

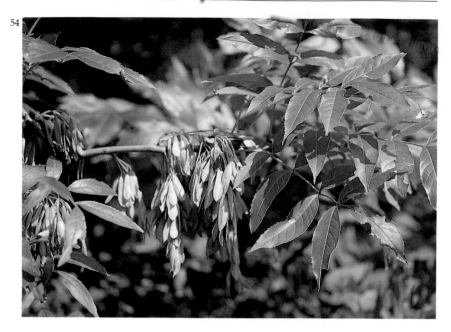

55

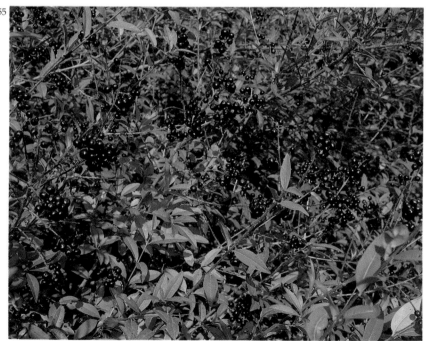

56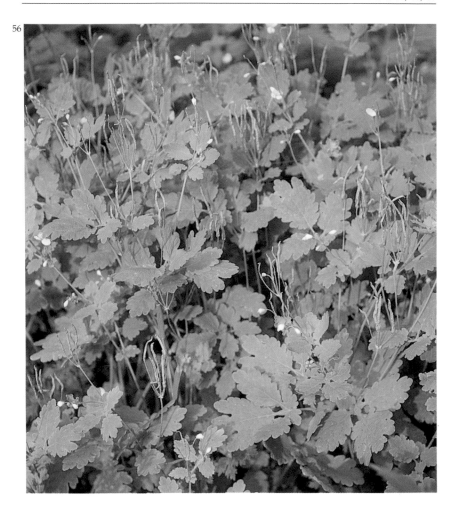

54   Ash *(Fraxinus excelsior)*
      HCB

55   Privet *(Ligustrum vulgare)*
      A-Z

56   Greater Celandine
      (Chelidonium majus)
      HCB

57

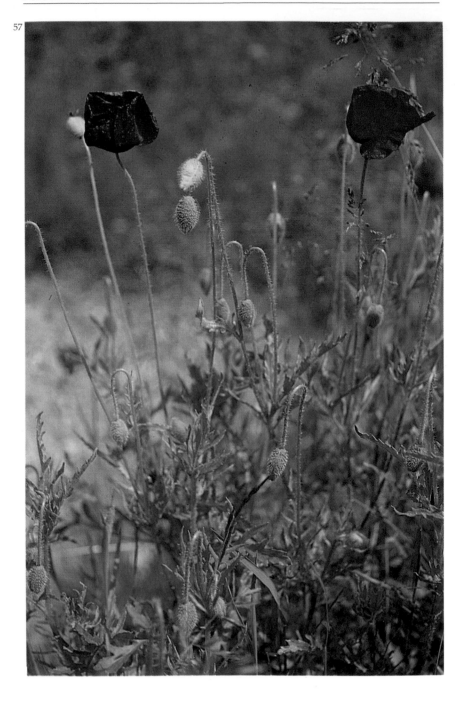

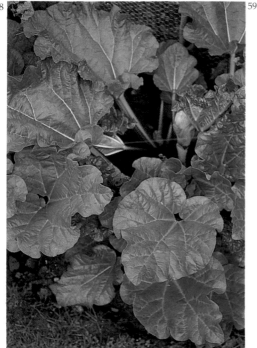

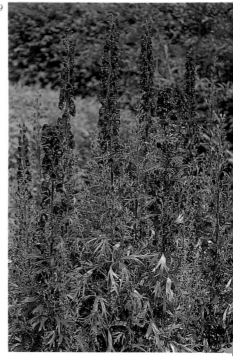

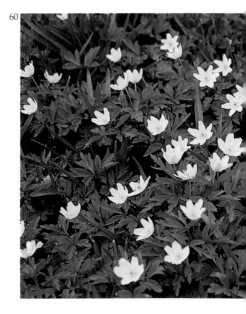

57   Field Poppy *(Papaver rhoeas)*
HCB

58   Rhubarb *(Rheum rhaponticum)*
HCB

59   Monkshood *(Aconitum napellus)*
HCB

60   Wood Anemone *(Anemone nemorosa)*
HCB

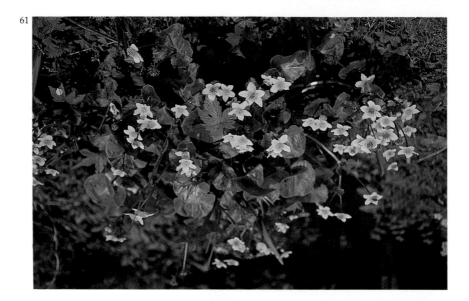

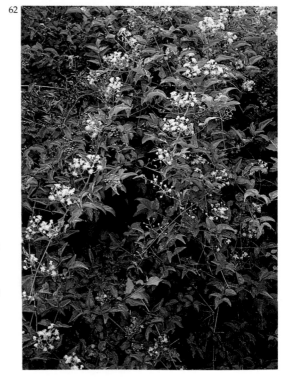

61 Marsh Marigold *(Caltha palustris)*
    HCB

62 Traveller's Joy *(Clematis vitalba)*
    HCB

63 Buttercup *(Ranunculus species)*
    HCB

63

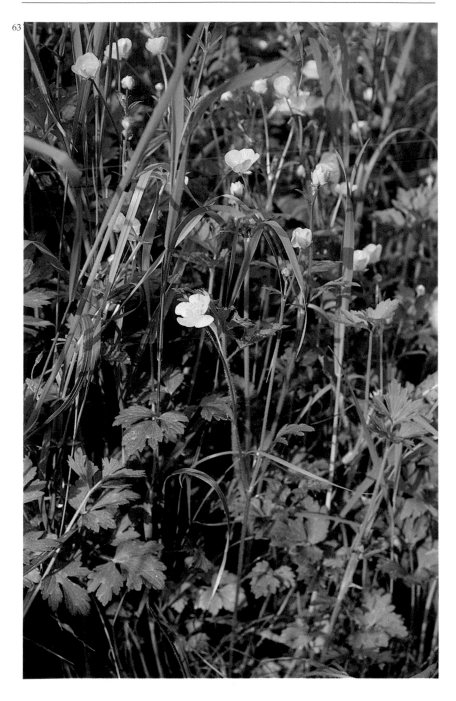

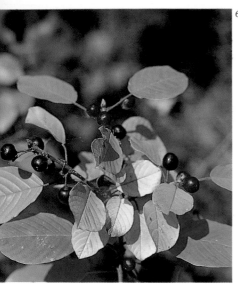

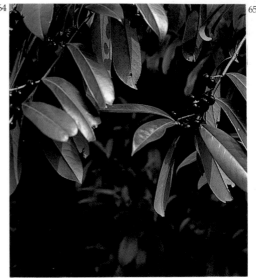

64   Buckthorn *(Rhamnus cathartica)*
      HCB

65   Cherry Laurel *(Prunus laurocerasus)*
      HCB

66   Foxglove *(Digitalis purpurea)*
      HCB

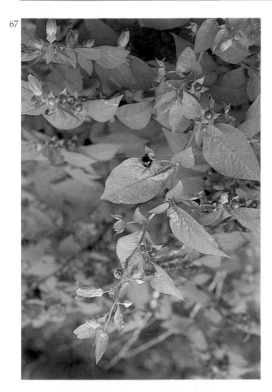

67 Deadly Nightshade
   (Atropa belladonna)
   HCB

68 Thorn Apple *(Datura
   stramonium)*
   A-Z

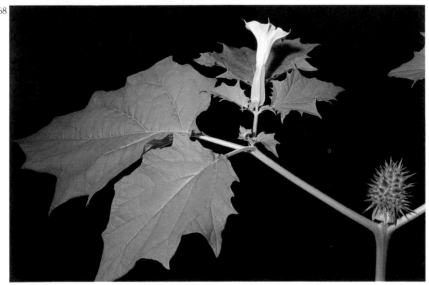

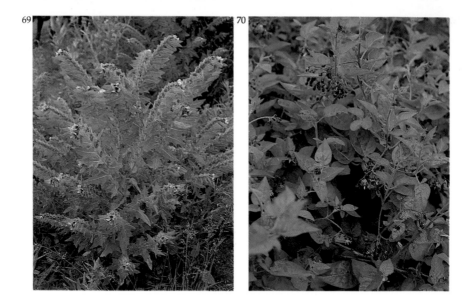

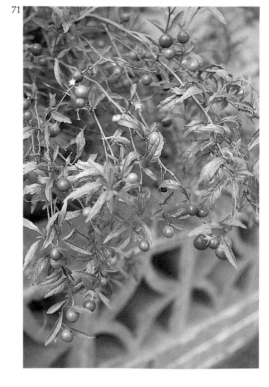

69 Henbane *(Hyoscyamus niger)*
HCB

70 Woody Nightshade *(Solanum dulcamara)*
HCB

71 Christmas Cherry *(Solanum pseudocapsicum)*
A-Z

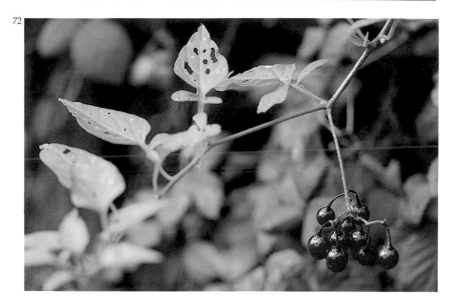

72   Woody Nightshade
    (Solanum dulcamara)
    HCB

73   Black Nightshade
    (Solanum nigrum)
    HCB

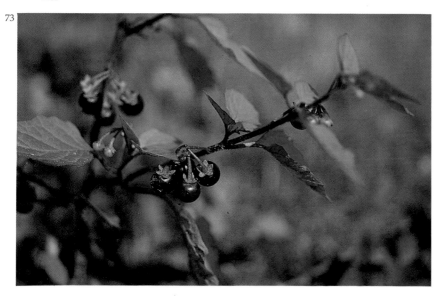

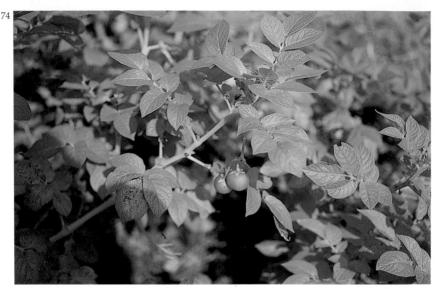

74   Potato *(Solanum tuberosum)*
      HCB

75   Yew *(Taxus baccata)*
      HCB

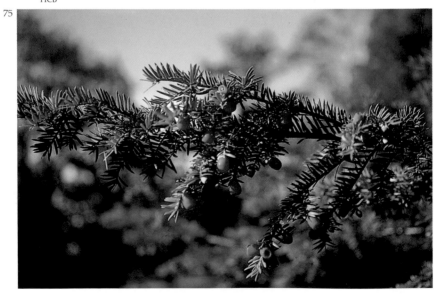

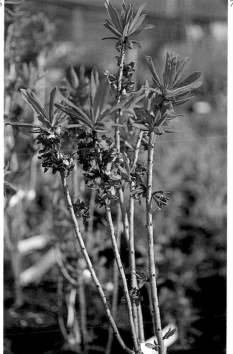

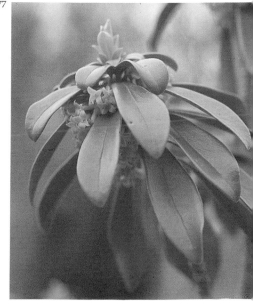

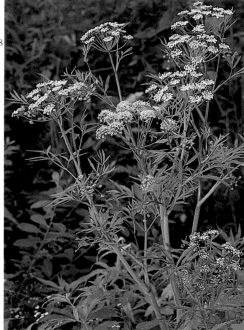

76   Mezereon *(Daphne mezereum)*
HCB

77   Spurge Laurel *(Daphne laureola)*
A-Z

78   Cowbane *(Cicuta virosa)*
AB

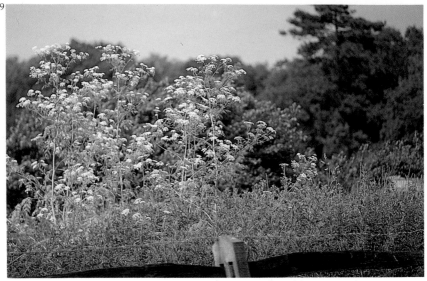

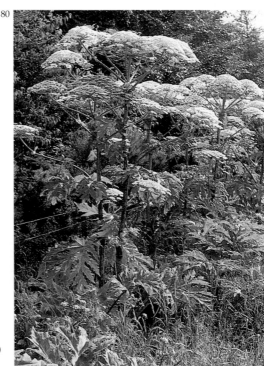

79   Hemlock (*Conium
      maculatum*)
      HCB

80   Giant Hogweed
      (*Heracleum mantegazzianum*)
      JCF

81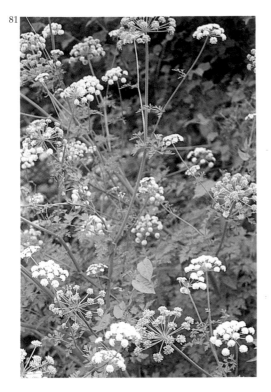

82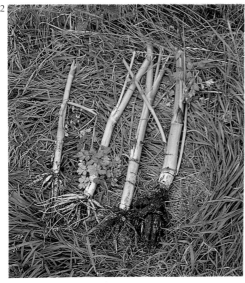

81   Hemlock Water Dropwort
      (Oenanthe crocata)
      HCB

82   Hemlock Water Dropwort
      (Oenanthe crocata)
      HCB

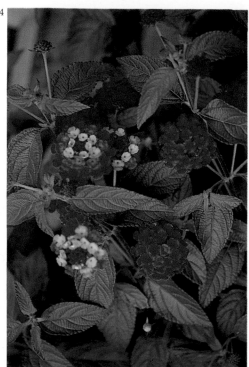

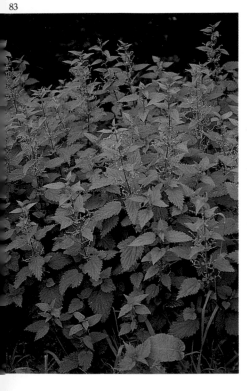

83 Stinging Nettle *(Urtica dioica)*
    HCB

84 Lantana *(Lantana camara)*
    HCB

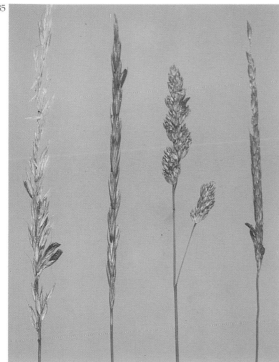

85 Ergot *(Claviceps* species) on wild grasses
ADAS

86 Death Cap *(Amanita phalloides)*
HCB

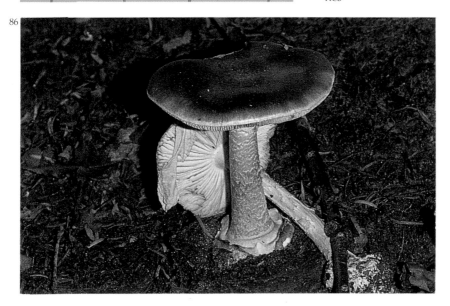

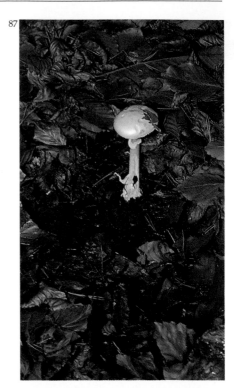

87   Destroying Angel
(Amanita virosa)
HCB

88   Cortinarius *(Cortinarius speciosissimus)*
DAR

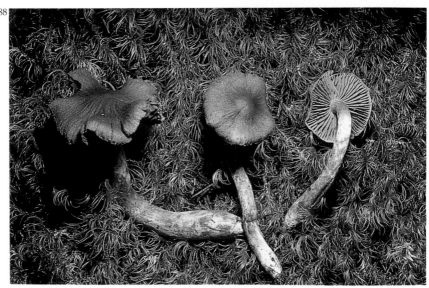

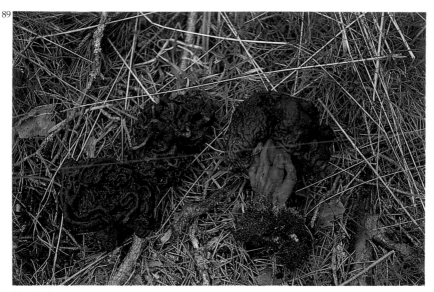

89   False Morel *(Gyromitra esculenta)*
DAR

90   Grey Mottle Gill *(Panaeolus sphinctrinus)*
RBG Edin

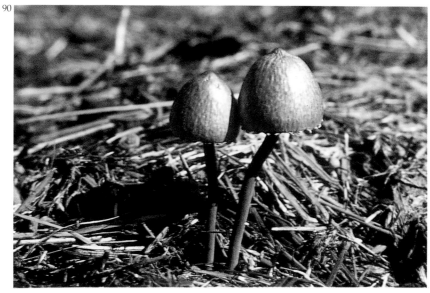

91

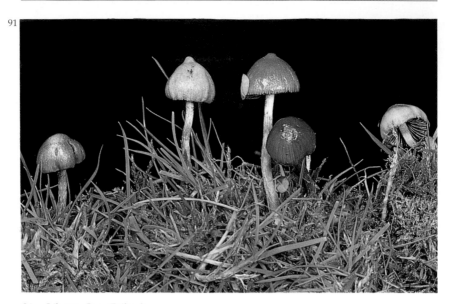

91 Liberty Cap *(Psilocybe
    semilanceata)*
    RBG Edin

92 Dung Roundhead
    (Stropharia semiglobata)
    RBG Edin

92

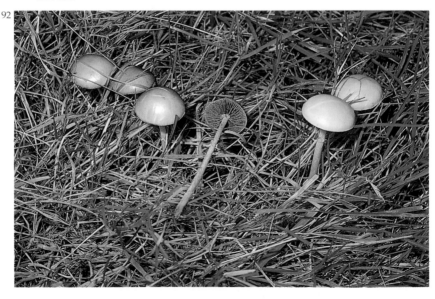

93

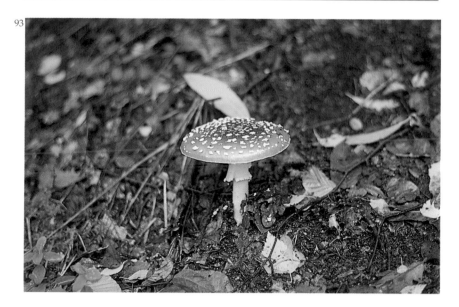

94

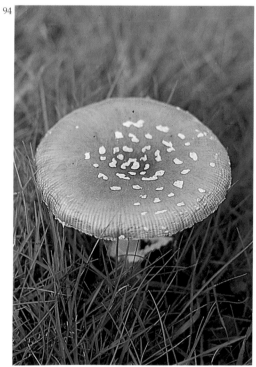

93 Fly Agaric *(Amanita muscaria)*
    HCB

94 Panther Cap *(Amanita pantherina)*
    HCB

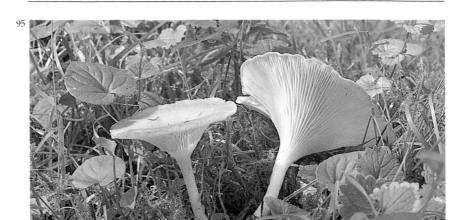

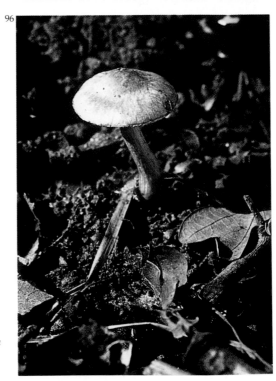

95   Clitocybe *(Clitocybe*
      species)*
      RBG Edin

96   Inocybe *(Inocybe geophylla*
      var *lilacina)*
      RBG Edin

97

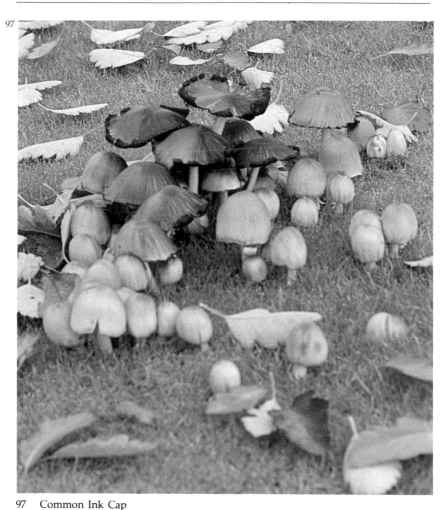

97 Common Ink Cap
    (Coprinus atramentarius)
    HCB

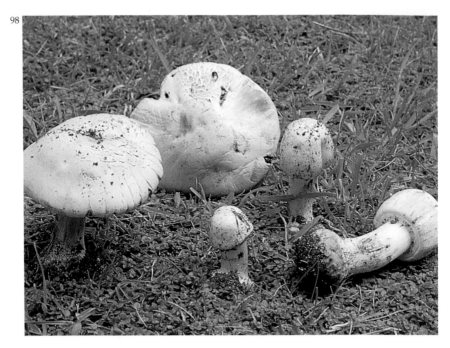

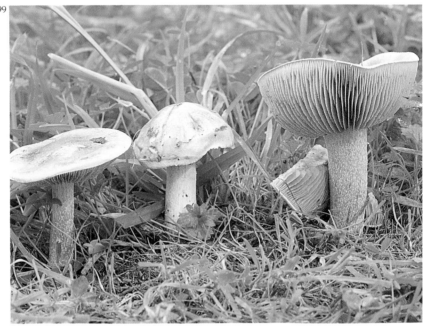

100

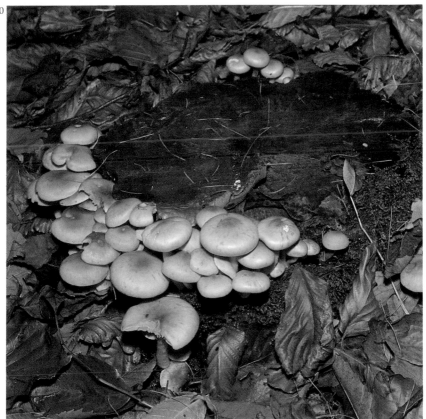

98 Yellow-Staining
    Mushroom *(Agaricus
    xanthodermus)*
    DAR

99 Fairy Cake Hebeloma
    (Hebeloma crustuliniforme)
    RBG Edin

100 Sulphur Tuft *(Hypholoma
    fasciculare)*
    HCB

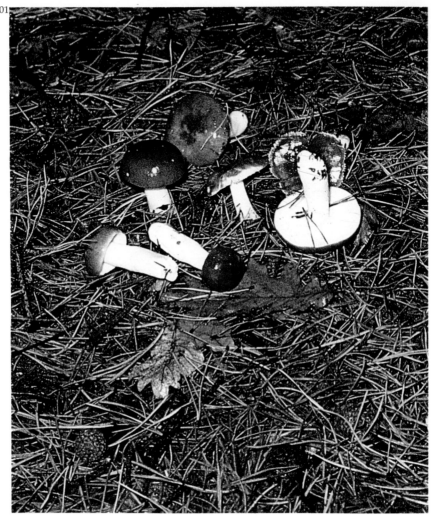

101 Sickener *(Russula emetica)*
HCB

Poisonous fungi

A few members of this large group can be fatally poisonous, some can cause severe or mild poisoning, some merely have an unpleasant taste but are otherwise harmless, while others are edible and have a delicious taste. It should be noted, however, that even edible fungi can cause poisoning if old or in poor condition when eaten. Identification, even with the aid of books, is not easy and great caution should therefore be exercised when contemplating eating any fungus; poisoning often results from incorrect identification. On the Continent, where collecting wild fungi to eat is a much more common practice than it is here, there is undoubtedly greater knowledge of the types of fungi that are edible, but there are also more cases of poisoning. Contrary to popular belief, there are no special characteristics by which an edible fungus can be recognized, and the names 'mushroom' and 'toadstool' (possibly related to the German 'Todesstuhl,' seat of death) give no indication of relative toxicity and can be used almost interchangeably.

There is little definite information available on the toxicity of fungi for animals except under experimental conditions. Farm animals usually avoid fungi, but domestic pets occasionally eat them and may be poisoned. It is said that deer can eat poisonous fungi with impunity.

The descriptions given here are intended only for guidance; for further details reference should be made to the many excellent, illustrated books available. Most of this section deals with the larger fungi (mushrooms and toadstools), but ergot, which is sometimes found in the ears of cereal crops, and mycotoxins, produced by some mould fungi in stored food and hay, are also included. The larger fungi have been grouped according to the type of poisoning they cause:

fungi causing cell damage   fungi containing muscarine
hallucinogenic fungi   fungi poisoning with alcohol
fungi containing ibotenic acid   fungi affecting only the digestive system

Within these groups the individual fungi are arranged alphabetically by their scientific (Latin) names. Brief information on some other poisonous fungi is given in the list on pages 124-125.

MYCOTOXINS

Some moulds that grow on foodstuffs produce toxins, very small amounts of which can cause human and animal poisoning. They are called mycotoxins, 'myco' being derived from the Greek word for a fungus. It is important to realize that not all moulds produce mycotoxins, and that mycotoxins may be present even when there is no obvious sign of moulds. Among the well-recognized mycotoxins that have caused disease are aflatoxin, ochratoxin and zearalenone. As their presence can be detected only be specialized analytical techniques, it is unwise to eat or give to animals any food that appears mouldy, whether it is fresh plant material, hay, grain, nuts, fruit or cooked products. In Britain there have been a few outbreaks of animal disease attributed to mycotoxins (mainly involving imported feed), but no cases of human poisoning have been reported. The effects of mycotoxins vary with the type of mould, the amount of mycotoxin present, and the animal species; they range from reduced growth rate to severe illness and death, with some specific mycotoxins inducing tumour formation, some affecting the reproductive organs and others the nervous system. It may well be that some plants are poisonous only because of their being infected by fungi, which produce mycotoxins, or which cause the plants themselves to produce anti-fungal substances that are also toxic to animals and man.

Apart from the possibility of mycotoxins being present, the use of mouldy feed and bedding materials for animals can present other dangers, as the spores of some moulds can give rise to allergic conditions affecting breathing (farmer's lung) in both animals and man.

ERGOT

Ergot *Claviceps* **species** (photo 85)

This fungus grows in the flowers of wild grasses and cereal crops, but is not usually recognized until the seed head or grain is formed in autumn. It then appears as hard, black or blackish-purple protrusions ('ergots'), replacing some of the grains and interspersed among them in the ear. These black masses are the resting stage of the fungus, and survive through the winter, after which the spores that develop within them germinate and infect new plants.

• POISONOUS SUBSTANCES Alkaloids are present in the ergot, the toxicity tending to decrease slowly during storage. The alkaloid content and consequently the toxicity of individual samples vary considerably.

• POISONING Ergotism (ergot poisoning) was not at all uncommon in the past in the human population of Europe, where it was caused by eating bread made from contaminated rye flour. Ergotized grass, hay and cereals have caused poisoning in horses, cattle, sheep, pigs and poultry. In both man and animals, two forms of the disease are recognized: a convulsive form with sudden onset that occurs when a large quantity of ergot is eaten in a short time, and a gangrenous form that develops slowly when small quantities are eaten over a long period. The convulsive form is characterized by loss of balance, staggering, trembling, numbness, cramps and convulsions; these are often preceded by digestive-system disturbances (vomiting and abdominal pain). The gangrenous form starts with tingling, pain, swelling, periods of extreme heat and cold, and then numbness in the extremities (hands, feet, tail and ears); dry gangrene can develop with loss of parts of these extremities. The stage with sensations of intense heat led to the disease being known in the Middle Ages as St. Anthony's fire.

The last outbreak of human ergotism in Britain was in Manchester in the late 1920s, but outbreaks in animals still occur occasionally, particularly in cattle in which the gangrenous form is more common.

• NOTE After being virtually absent from cereal crops in Britain for many years, ergot has become more prevalent since the late 1970s, particularly in Scotland. Ergot-infected wild grasses can act as reservoirs of infection for crops.

LARGER FUNGI

FUNGI CAUSING CELL DAMAGE

Death Cap *Amanita phalloides* (photo 86)

This dangerously poisonous fungus is fairly common in woods, especially beech and oak, in autumn. For the non-expert, it has no particularly striking, characteristic features and may be confused with other fungi. The smooth, moist cap is greenish yellow, darker at the centre, and faintly streaked radially. It is 6–12.5 cm (2½–5 in) across and easily peeled. The stalk is smooth, white and 6–12.5 cm (2½–5 in) high. There is an irregular ring near the top of the stalk and a bulbous cup at the base. The whole fungus has a sweetish smell.

• POISONOUS SUBSTANCES Amatoxins (cyclic octapeptides) are the cause of poisoning by this fungus; other toxic substances, including phallotoxins, are present, but are thought to be inactive in the digestive system and are therefore not involved in the toxic reaction that occurs when the fungus is eaten.

• POISONING This is one of the most poisonous fungi known; eating as little as half a cap can be fatal. Symptoms appear in two phases, separated by a period of apparent recovery which can be very misleading. In the first phase the digestive system is affected, with symptoms appearing in 6–24 hours; these include dryness of the mouth, vomiting, abdominal pain and diarrhoea, often with blood. These initial symptoms can be very severe, and last as long as 24 hours, after which they subside, and for up to three days it can appear that the patient has recovered. During this period, however, severe liver and kidney damage is taking place. Further symptoms then become apparent, with weakness, jaundice and general deterioration often culminating in delirium, convulsions, unconsciousness, and death.

Poisoning has occurred under natural conditions in goats, and experimentally in dogs, but in general little is known about the effects of this fungus on domestic animals.

Medical treatment is required urgently, as it is effective only in the early stages, before irreversible liver and kidney damage occurs.

● NOTE This fungus is extremely dangerous; even very small quantities can cause death.

Cortinarius *Cortinarius* species (photo 88)

Although many *Cortinarius* species are edible, a few are dangerously poisonous. These include *Cortinarius speciosissimus* and *C. gentilis* which are found mainly in coniferous woods in northern England and Scotland, and *C. orellanus* and *C. orellanoides*, found in deciduous woods further south. These fungi have generally been considered uncommon, but since their extremely poisonous nature was discovered recently, when there were some fatalities, the fungi have been identified more often. It is probable that they were present previously but had not been identified because of their close similarity to some other fungi.

Cortinarius speciosissimus is a brownish-orange fungus, having a cap up to 7.5 cm (3 in) across, with a central point and widely spaced, thick gills beneath. The stalk, 5–10 cm (2–4 in) high, is a similar colour but may have yellow bands. The other poisonous species are also a rusty brown or cinnamon colour. The flesh is yellowish-brown and is said to smell strongly of radish.

● POISONOUS SUBSTANCES These are cyclopeptides, one or a mixture of which has been called orellanin after *Cortinarius orellanus.*

● POISONING These fungi can cause fatal poisoning or such severe kidney damage that transplants may be needed. A characteristic feature of *Cortinarius* poisoning is the long delay of two to seventeen days before symptoms appear. Initially these are nausea and vomiting, followed by sweating, trembling, muscular and abdominal pains and great thirst; there may be constipation or diarrhoea. The kidneys are the main organs affected, with urine production decreased at first and then increased. As poisoning progresses, liver function is also affected, and sleepiness and convulsions develop. Death has occurred despite intensive treatment in hospital. Many incidents have been reported on the Continent, and in 1979, three people were poisoned by *Cortinarius speciosissimus* in Scotland; two had to have kidney transplants.

No information is available on the toxicity of these fungi for domestic animals.

The severity of *Cortinarius* poisoning necessitates hospital treatment; medical advice should be sought urgently if poisoning is suspected, and not delayed until symptoms develop, when irreversible damage to the kidneys and liver may already have taken place.

• NOTE These fungi are extremely dangerous and can cause fatal poisoning. All orange and reddish-brown fungi of this type should be avoided unless positively identified as edible species.

False Morel *Gyromitra esculenta* (photo 89)

This fungus may be found in coniferous woods in spring. It is uncommon in Britain. The cap is irregularly grooved and folded and is chestnut brown in colour. It is up to 10 cm (4 in) high and 15 cm (6 in) wide at its widest point. The stalk is thick and grooved, grey or pinkish in colour and about 6 cm (2½ in) high.

• POISONOUS SUBSTANCE The fungus contains gyromitrin from which the toxic substance monomethylhydrazine is liberated. The latter, and related compounds, have been used as fuel for rockets and space craft; because of this their toxic properties have been studied in considerable detail.

• POISONING False morel has been grown commercially on the Continent, as it appeared to be safe to eat after drying or boiling for at least ten minutes; the fresh or lightly cooked fungus has, however, caused serious poisoning as a result of damage to the liver, kidneys and other organs. The vapour given off during cooking has also caused poisoning. The first symptoms generally appear about six hours after eating the fungi but have been reported several hours earlier or later than this. Digestive-system disturbances, including nausea, repeated vomiting, stomach ache and diarrhoea, are followed by weakness, dizziness and unsteadiness. Up to five days later there may also be jaundice, breathing problems, convulsions and coma in severe cases; sometimes the poisoning is fatal.

Medical advice should be sought.

HALLUCINOGENIC FUNGI

There are several fungi in this group, related only by their hallucinatory effects when eaten, and not by any obvious visible similarities. These fungi have been given many common names, reflecting their properties. Among those most often used are magic mushrooms, laughing mushrooms, happy mushrooms and sillys.

Gymnopilus species

These have orange or tan-coloured caps, up to 12.5 cm (5 in) across, covered with minute, radiating fibres; some have small scales on the surface, and some a central 'boss'. The stalks are the same colour or paler than the caps, and may be thick and fibrous, or slender, depending on the species. Some *Gymnopilus* species grow in tufts on or near tree stumps, where they could be confused with the superficially similar honey fungus (*Armillaria mellea*), which is edible. Poisoning, see below.

Mower's Mushroom *Panaeolina foenisecii*

This small fungus is very common on lawns and in cut grass from early summer to autumn. The cap is a dull, slightly reddish brown and is bell shaped or convex, and 1–2 cm (⅓–¾ in) across; when dry it becomes paler from the centre outwards. The gills are mottled brown, and the stalk is slender and delicate, up to 6 cm (2½ in) high. Poisoning, see below.

Panaeolus subbalteatus

Tufts of these small fungi are commonly found on recently manured ground. The caps, up to 4 cm (1½ in) across, are pale brown, darker when moist. They are convex initially, but often have upturned edges when older. The stalk is slender, paler than the cap and up to 7.5 cm (3 in) high. The gills beneath the cap are closely crowded and mottled dark brown. Other *Panaeolus* species, including grey mottle gill (*Panaeolus sphinctrinus*, photo 90), also have hallucinogenic properties. Poisoning, see below.

Psilocybe species (photo 91)

The poisonous substance, psilocybin, was named after these fungi but, due to the re-naming of several of them, there are only a few still bearing the name. The best known hallucinogenic fungus in the group is the liberty cap (*Psilocybe semilanceata*). It occurs in small groups in grassland and heath, and is common throughout the country. The cap, usually less than 1 cm (⅓ in) across, is light brown and conical, with an incurved, often slightly split and ragged margin. The gills are brownish purple or black, with white edges. The stalks are slender, paler than the cap, up to 7.5 cm (3 in) high, and often irregularly wavy. Poisoning, see below.

Dung Roundhead *Stropharia semiglobata* (photo 92)

This small, common fungus can be found at all times of year growing, usually in groups, on dung or recently manured ground. The caps are smooth, slimy domes, 1-4 cm (⅓-1½ in) across, and pale yellow or straw coloured. Initially the gills are purplish brown, but become almost black as the spores mature. The thin stalks are up to 10 cm (4 in) high, white or paler yellow than the cap, except for a thin, dark ring near the top.

• **POISONOUS SUBSTANCES** These fungi contain the hallucinogenic indole psilocybin and possibly very small amounts of psilocin. Psilocybin remains active for many years in dried fungal material. When the fungi are eaten, some psilocybin is converted to psilocin, an even more powerful hallucinogenic agent. There is considerable variation in the hallucinogen content of these fungi.

• **POISONING** As their many common names imply, these fungi are known for their psychoactive properties and ability to produce psychedelic effects similar to those of the drug LSD; they are therefore grown and eaten deliberately, often in quite large numbers. Both pleasant and unpleasant reactions may be experienced. Effects such as feelings of well-being and relaxation, sharpened perception of colours and outlines of objects, and the appearance of brightly coloured, rapidly changing patterns when the eyes are closed, start within half an hour and continue for up to three hours after eating the mushrooms or drinking liquid in which they have been cooked. Undesired effects can also occur: nausea, vomiting, abdominal pain, diarrhoea, rapid breathing, headache, tension, anxiety, dizziness, confusion, agitation, panic, and delirium with uncontrollable laughter. In addition there is the risk of accidents occurring as the result of abnormal or dangerous behaviour while hallucinating. Full recovery can be expected within 18 hours, although there are reports of more severe cases that have taken longer. The most dangerous aspect of collecting these fungi is the possibility of confusing them with similar, rather nondescript fungi that could be dangerously poisonous, such as some *Galerina* species (see list, page 124).

The only treatment usually required is rest and reassurance in a quiet environment, with continuous observation to prevent accidents.

FUNGI CONTAINING IBOTENIC ACID

Fly Agaric *Amanita muscaria* (photo 93)

This is probably one of the best known fungi in Britain as it is so easily recognized; it is often illustrated in wildlife paintings and children's books. It grows beneath trees, usually birch, in light shade, in summer and autumn. When young, the cap is a bright-red sphere with numerous white wart-like patches. It expands to become flat or slightly convex, up to 15 cm (6 in) across, with more white patches towards the edges than at the centre; with age the characteristic red fades to orange. The stalk is white and has a bulbous base and a white ring near the top. Poisoning, see below.

Panther Cap *Amanita pantherina* (photo 94)

This fungus is similar to fly agaric, but usually grows at the edge of beech woods. The cap is smaller, up to 7.5 cm (3 in) across, and is olive green to brown in colour, with white wart-like patches.

● **POISONOUS SUBSTANCES** These fungi contain ibotenic acid which is readily converted to muscimol, a more potent toxin; individual fungi vary in the amount they contain. Muscarine, the principal toxin of some *Clitocybe* and *Inocybe* species, is also present but in insufficient quantities to cause poisoning.

● **POISONING** The reputation of these fungi for being deadly poisonous is probably unjustified. Although severe symptoms can arise, complete recovery generally follows. Within an hour or so of eating the fungi, there is drowsiness, dizziness and sometimes digestive-system symptoms and loss of muscular coordination. These are accompanied by elation and excitability, with mental and visual aberrations but not true hallucinations. A characteristic feature is a deep sleep that may develop into coma. The major effects usually subside within eight hours.

Similar symptoms have been caused in dogs and cats by both of the fungi; paralysis of the legs has also been reported in dogs.

Professional advice should be sought in all but the mildest cases. In treating poisoning by these fungi, it is important not to use atropine (a specific antidote for muscarine) as this increases the adverse effects of ibotenic acid.

FUNGI CONTAINING MUSCARINE

Clitocybe species (photo 95)

These are rather fleshy fungi, mainly dull in colour, and characterized by the gills extending down the top of the stalk, and the indented centre of the cap, giving a funnel shape, sometimes with a small raised 'boss' in the middle. It is important to identify these fungi correctly because some of the smaller, dangerously poisonous ones, with caps up to 5 cm (2 in) across, resemble, and often grow with, the edible fairy ring fungus (*Marasmius oreades*). Poisoning, see below.

Inocybe species (photo 96)

Correct identification of these fungi can sometimes be achieved only with the aid of a microscope, so it would be advisable to avoid eating any of them because some are dangerously poisonous. A convex cap generally less than 5 cm (2 in) across, with minute radiating fibres and a central 'boss', is typical of *Inocybe*; many are brownish, but a few are pale mauve or pinkish.

• POISONOUS SUBSTANCE These fungi contain a quarternary ammonium compound called muscarine, after the fly agaric (*Amanita muscaria*), in which it was first found, but which, in fact, contains very little muscarine. Muscarine remains active after the fungi are cooked.

• POISONING Symptoms usually appear about 15–30 minutes after eating these fungi. A combination of three symptoms is characteristic of muscarine poisoning: excessive production of sweat, saliva and tears, known as the PSL syndrome (perspiration, salivation and lacrimation). Nausea, vomiting and abdominal pain are also common, and if sufficient quantities are eaten there may be blurred vision with contracted pupils, slow heart beat, wheezing, dizziness and diarrhoea.

Domestic animals rarely eat fungi, but the potential danger of some of them is demonstrated in the case of a dog which ate *Clitocybe* species, and became unsteady in its movements and produced a clear frothy fluid before vomiting several times and having diarrhoea; it had recovered about two hours later. Some *Clitocybe* species smell of aniseed, which is attractive to dogs.

As there have been a few fatal cases, professional advice should be sought unless the symptoms are only very mild. For treatment there is a specific antidote, atropine, the dosage of which can be decided by the doctor on the basis of the severity of symptoms. It should be noted, however, that it is

119

dangerous to use this muscarine antidote for poisoning by *Amanita muscaria*, the activity of whose toxin (ibotenic acid) is increased by atropine.

FUNGI POISONOUS WITH ALCOHOL

Common Ink Cap *Coprinus atramentarius*
(photo 97)

This fungus is common in autumn, but can be seen occasionally throughout the year. It is usually found in small groups near tree stumps, but may also be found in fields or gardens. The cap is ribbed radially, greyish brown, darker and slightly scaly towards the centre; initially it is shaped like a wide bell, up to 7·5 cm (3 in) high, but expands and flattens as it matures. Finally the edge of the cap becomes ragged and moist and gradually disintegrates into black inky drops containing the spores. The stalk is also greyish, often paler than the cap and up to 20 cm (8 in) high, tapering upwards from the base where there is a clearly visible, white, ring-like zone.

● POISONOUS SUBSTANCE This fungus contains a compound named coprine that causes poisoning only in the presence of alcohol, and has a similar mode of action to the drug Antabuse (disulfiram) used in the treatment of alcoholism. The effect is the same whether the fungus is eaten raw or cooked.

● POISONING In the absence of alcohol, the common ink cap is edible, but if alcohol has been taken a few hours before to a few days after eating it, signs of poisoning can occur. There are considerable differences in the sensitivity of individuals to this type of poisoning. Within half an hour there is flushing of the face and neck, then a rapid, throbbing pulse, dizziness, perspiration and tingling of the fingers. Nausea, vomiting, headache and, occasionally, mental confusion may be experienced. The symptoms usually subside, without treatment, in three or four hours but may recur if more alcohol is taken.

FUNGI AFFECTING ONLY THE DIGESTIVE SYSTEM

These fungi are grouped together because they all cause relatively mild, digestive-system disturbances and generally no other symptoms; most are unrelated and dissimilar in appearance.

Yellow-Staining Mushroom
Agaricus xanthodermus (photo 98)

This fungus is fairly common in late summer and autumn, often growing in groups in leaf mould or compost in pastures, woodland and gardens. The cap is 6–12·5 cm (2½–5 in) across, generally smooth and white except for a few fine scales near the centre; the edge often splits and cracks when mature. The gills are pinkish at first, then brown. The stalk is also white, up to 12·5 cm (5 in) high, with a fleshy white ring near the top. The flesh of both the cap and the stalk become bright yellow when bruised or scratched.

Especially when young, this species can easily be confused with the edible horse mushroom (*Agaricus arvensis*), the flesh of which also turns yellow when bruised. The two can be readily distinguished, however, because the flesh of the slightly thickened base of the stalk is a vivid yellow in the yellow-staining mushroom, and it has an unpleasant smell, rather like ink, that is particularly noticeable during cooking. Poisoning, see below.

Devil's Boletus *Boletus satanas*

This is a rare fungus that grows in autumn, beneath deciduous trees on chalky soils. It is sturdy, with a thick, domed cap 10–30 cm (4–12 in) across. It is pale grey at first, but brownish when older. The tubes beneath the cap are yellow inside, but the visible openings (pores) are usually red. The stalk is yellowish with a network of red veins near the cap, but red and greatly swollen at the base.

It is poisonous, causing persistent vomiting when raw, but is harmless, although unpleasant in taste, when thoroughly cooked.

Livid Entoloma *Entoloma sinuatum*

This fungus, that grows in parks and gardens in early autumn, is still sometimes referred to by its old name *Entoloma lividum*. It is a thick, fleshy fungus with a light-grey cap that becomes tinged with yellow. The edge of the cap is wavy and the surface may have irregular, rounded undulations. When fully grown the cap is up to 15 cm (6 in) across, and the thick, greyish or pale yellow stalk is up to 10 cm (4 in) high. At first the gills are yellow but become pinkish as the pink spores develop. Poisoning, see below.

Fairy Cake Hebeloma *Hebeloma crustuliniforme*
(photo 99)

In autumn, this fungus is fairly common in deciduous woods and sometimes grows on heathland. The cap, usually less than 7·5 cm (3 in) across, is domed in young specimens but flattens and often has a slightly undulating edge when old. It is slightly sticky, pale biscuit coloured or light tan, but dark droplets from the greyish-brown gills hang from its edge in damp weather and tend to leave dark marks when dry. The stalk is usually about 5 cm (2 in) high and is whitish, with small scales on the upper part. The whole fungus smells of radish. Poisoning, see below.

Sulphur Tuft *Hypholoma fasciculare* (photo 100)

This very common fungus grows in crowded clumps at the base of tree stumps and is particularly abundant in autumn. The cap is domed at first, but expands to a shallow bell shape, up to 5 cm (2 in) across, as it grows. It is a bright sulphur yellow with a tan colour near the apex. The stalk is also yellow, sometimes tan coloured at the base; it is 5–15 cm (2–6 in) high and often slightly curved. The gills beneath the cap are yellow at first but become olive green or brownish as the spores mature. Poisoning, see below.

Sickener *Russula emetica* (photo 101)

This common autumn fungus grows beneath coniferous trees, often in moss. The cap, up to 10 cm (4 in) across, is smooth, moist and uniformly bright red or pinkish red. It is dome shaped initially but often with upturned edges and a depressed centre later. The gills are white. The stalk is white and usually longer than the diameter of the cap. The sickener has a hot, acrid taste and causes vomiting if eaten raw. Some other *Russula* species, such as *Russula fellea* and *Russula nauseosa*, have similar effects.

• POISONOUS SUBSTANCES Little is known about the agents responsible for this type of poisoning. There is often considerable variation in the amount of toxin present in these fungi if growing in different locations or even in the same location in different seasons. Some are harmful only when raw and others only when old.

• POISONING The susceptibility of individuals to some of these fungi also varies considerably. Symptoms usually appear within two hours of eating the fungi. Nausea, vomiting, abdominal pain and diarrhoea are commonly experienced, although not all of these necessarily occur in each case. Other symptoms that occur occasionally are headache, dizziness, difficult breathing and unconsciousness. *Agaricus xanthodermus* (page 121) and *Entoloma sinuatum* (page 121) are more likely to cause serious poisoning than the others.

Recovery usually occurs within 24 hours, but, if symptoms are severe or persist, medical advice should be sought.

• NOTE As poisoning by some of the most dangerous fungi often starts with digestive upsets, it is most important to identify correctly the fungi responsible for the symptoms. If in doubt, professional advice should be sought urgently.

Other poisonous fungi

An annotated list

Unless positively identified, all fungi should be treated with caution. This list includes most of the fungi of lesser importance that are likely to cause poisoning in Britain; the more important ones are described in the main section of the text (pages 113–123).

The fungi are listed alphabetically by their scientific (Latin) names.

Fungus	Type of poisoning
Woodland Yellow Stainer *Agaricus placomyces*	Can cause digestive-system disturbances.
Wood Mushroom *Agaricus silvicola*	Can cause digestive-system disturbances.
Fool's Mushroom, Deadly Agaric *Amanita verna*	Resembles death cap (page 113) but uniformly white and rare in Britain. Poisoning similar and can be fatal. Cattle have been poisoned.
Destroying Angel *Amanita virosa*	Resembles death cap (page 113) but uniformly white. Poisoning similar and can be fatal. Photo 87.
Club-Foot Mushroom *Clitocybe clavipes*	Poisonous with alcohol, similar to common ink cap poisoning (page 120).
Conocybe *Conocybe* species	Some contain similar toxins to death cap (page 113) but are far less poisonous.
Galerina *Galerina* species	Some contain similar toxins to death cap (page 113) but are less poisonous.
Milk Caps *Lactarius* species	Some may cause vomiting and diarrhoea.
Stinking Parasol *Lepiota cristata*	Contains similar toxins to death cap (page 113) but is far less poisonous.
Copper Trumpet *Omphalotus olearius*	Contains muscarine (page 119). Very rare in Britain.

Fungus	Type of poisoning
Roll Rim *Paxillus involutus*	May cause digestive-system disturbances if eaten raw.
Shaggy Pholiota *Pholiota squarrosa*	Can cause mild digestive-system disturbances.
Handsome Clavaria *Ramaria formosa*	Can cause digestive-system disturbances.
Earthballs *Scleroderma* species	Some may cause abdominal pain, nausea, and vomiting.
Verdigris Agaric *Stropharia aeruginosa*	Sometimes causes digestive-system disturbances.
Tricholoma *Tricholoma* species	Some are edible, some cause digestive-system disturbances, muscular weakness and loss of coordination. Careful identification is essential.

Index

Printed in the United Kingdom for Her Majesty's Stationery Office
Dd 239593   C 50   3/88